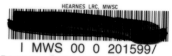
Studies in Disorders of Communication

General Editors:

Professor David Crystal
Honorary Professor of Linguistics, University College of North Wales,
Bangor

Professor Ruth Lesser
University of Newcastle upon Tyne

Professor Margaret Snowling
University of Newcastle upon Tyne

D0988703

Psychogenic Voice Disorders and Cognitive–Behaviour Therapy

Peter Butcher
Department of Psychology
The Royal London Hospital

Annie Elias
Department of Speech and Language Therapy
Kent and Canterbury Hospital

Ruth Raven
Department of Speech and Language Therapy
The General Infirmary at Leeds

With a contribution from Jenny Yeatman,
The Royal London Hospital

Foreword by Professor Arnold Aronson
Professor of Speech Pathology, Mayo Clinic and Mayo Foundation,
Rochester, MN, USA

SINGULAR PUBLISHING GROUP, INC.
SAN DIEGO, CALIFORNIA

© 1993 Whurr Publishers Ltd
19b Compton Terrace, London N1 2UN, England
Published and distributed in the USA and Canada by
SINGULAR PUBLISHING GROUP, INC.
4284 41st Street
San Diego, California 92105

British Library Cataloguing-in-Publication Data
A catalogue record for this book is available from the
British Library.

ISBN 1-870332-20-6

Library of Congress Cataloging-in-Publication Data
A catalogue record for this book is available.
Singular number 1-56593-238-2

Photoset by Stephen Cary
Printed and bound in the UK by Athenaeum Press Ltd,
Newcastle upon Tyne

Foreword

This book, which is devoted to the diagnosis and treatment of psychogenic voice disorders, is long overdue. It has taken far too long for specialists in voice disorders to acknowledge that most so-called 'functional', or non-organic, voice disorders are caused primarily by different degrees and types of psychological disturbances. Throughout the decades over which voice disorders have grown into a subspecialty, we have witnessed patients whose laryngeal examinations are normal but who are mute, aphonic, breathy, hoarse, have falsetto pitch breaks or excessively high pitch. Although we have no statistics as to how many of these patients received serious, probing, psychosocial interviews, there is much empirical evidence that in most of these patients such investigation is consistently omitted. It has been my perception over the years that the reason for this omission can be laid at the doorsteps of our educational institutions, which fail to include training in psychosocial interviewing and psychotherapy as part of their speech pathology curricula. When a student does emerge from the university with such a background, it would appear to have been by mere chance that he or she had a professor who personally saw the necessity for such education or that the student realised the need and pursued psychological training individually. Such haphazard preparation is no longer acceptable. It is paradoxical that, as a profession, we are quick to pick up on the latest computers, diagnostic and therapeutic instrumentation, and tests and measures, no matter how intricate, and yet we will neglect teaching students the fundamentals of how to relate to human beings whose communicative disorders are often caused by personal problems, or whose personal problems are often caused by their communicative disorders, and who need someone with whom they can discuss the emotional implications of their voice disorders.

Why is it taking us so long to acknowledge and to deal more effectively with these voice disorders despite incontestable evidence that they are of emotional origin? I believe that there is a multiple answer to this question. We are afraid to elicit emotions in our patients. In fact, we are not even trained to deal effectively with our own emotions. We are reluctant to encroach upon what we believe is alien territory. We conjecture, incorrectly, that if we let the psychological genie out of the bottle, it may be harmful to us and the patient. The result of these attitudes is that no-one appears willing to take the responsibility for investigating and treating the patient whose voice disorder is a direct result of acute or chronic emotional conflict. Instead of facing this important responsibility, we continue to perpetuate old practices, which, although they have their place, are too often ineffectual by themselves. So we just keep using the old cookbook recipes of breathing exercises, optimum pitch training, biofeedback and relaxation.

During 30 years of dealing with patients referred for the investigation of voice disorders, I have found it a rare occurrence for anyone outside speech pathology to take the time to perform a diagnostic psychosocial interview. The otolaryngologist does not do this for reasons of insufficient time, training and inclination. The same can be said for internists and general practitioners. Yet, the psychosocial history is not only crucial for diagnosis; it cannot be gracefully separated from symptomatic voice therapy which often has to accompany the externalisation of emotions.

If speech pathologists are to expand into the realm of patient psychological interviewing, we will have to become convinced, through personal experience, that the psychological life of the patient is directly responsible for the voice disorder. But, if we are untrained to ask, and if, as is usually the case with psychogenic voice patients, they do not voluntarily disclose psychologically pertinent information, examiner and patient will continue to saunter blithely down the path, oblivious to the critical core of the voice problem.

For these reasons, one finds it heartening that a book such as this recognises the validity of the connection between disturbed lives and abnormal voices. But, it goes one important step further – by advocating that speech–language pathologists can, and need, to learn how to administer psychosocial interviewing as well as psychological therapy as a means of effecting total care for the voice-disordered patient. The idea of psychological therapy is a quantum leap in the advocacy of greater responsibilities for members of our profession. Importantly, there is a scientific basis for such advocacy which can be found in the research of Peter Butcher and his colleagues in the UK. This shows that, in collaboration with a psychologist or cognitive–behaviour therapist, speech pathologists can safely and effectively administer psychotherapy to voice patients.

The obstacle that we now face is not of proving that psychological stress and interpersonal conflict are pivotal causes of voice disorders and that the treatment of such causes often leads to alleviation of the voice disorder; ample literature establishes this connection beyond a reasonable doubt. Rather, what challenges us today is convincing educational authorities of the reality and validity of psychogenic voice disturbances and to persuade them that they need to expand their curricula to include education in the psychological and psychiatric aspects of voice disorders. Make no mistake about it, this is not an easy area to learn. It is antithetical to mechanistic, rigid, procedurally oriented therapy. It requires education and training in the theory of somatisation and conversion disorders and, in practice, how to behave and to think like a clinical psychologist or psychiatrist. We have to be prepared to be the first to ask patients questions about psychological causes of their voice disorders, and to be prepared for patient resistance, denial and even anger in response to such questions. We have to learn to draw upon our own stability so that we can deal unflinchingly with the entire spectrum of emotional responses in patients, ranging from denial through grief to anger. We must be prepared to confront failure when patients unyieldingly deny that they have any problems whatsoever.

If we are willing to acknowledge the above and to train our students appropriately and adequately in psychogenic voice disorders, the rewards will be not only a feeling of accomplishment on our part but also a feeling of providing a more effective service to the voice-disordered population. For, there will occur a reduction in the incidence of misdiagnosis and an increase in the percentage of patients cured or significantly helped in a much shorter period of time than taken by the symptomatic voice therapy which often grinds on for weeks or months with little or no benefit to the patient. One hopes that this book will speed us to that desired objective.

Arnold E. Aronson, PhD
March 1993

General preface

This series focuses upon disorders of speech language and communication, bringing together the techniques of analysis, assessment and treatment which are pertinent to the area. It aims to cover cognitive, linguistic, social and education aspects of language disability, and therefore has relevance within a number of disciplines. These include speech therapy, the education of children and adults with special needs, teachers of the deaf, teachers of English as a second language and of foreign languages, and educational and clinical psychology. The research and clinical findings from these various areas can usefully inform one another and, therefore, we hope one of the main functions of this series will be to put people within one profession in touch with developments in another. Thus, it is our editorial policy to ask authors to consider the implications of their findings for professions outside their own and for fields with which they have not been primarily concerned. We hope to engender an integrated approach to theory and practice and to produce a much-needed emphasis on the description and analysis of language as such, as well as on the provision of specific techniques of therapy, remediation and rehabilitation

Whilst it has been our aim to restrict the series to the study of language disability, its scope goes considerably beyond this. Many previously neglected topics have been included where these seem to benefit from contemporary research in linguistics, psychology, medicine, sociology, education and English studies. Each volume puts its subject matter in perspective and provides an introductory slant to its presentation. In this way we hope to provide specialised studies which can be used as texts for components of teaching courses at undergraduate and postgraduate levels, as well as material directly applicable to the needs of professional workers.

David Crystal
Ruth Lesser
Margaret Snowling

Preface

In the last decade there has been significant international interest in voice disorders. This has resulted in a greater understanding of the voice together with an expansion of the literature, and it has been an exciting field in which to work. In the UK this is reflected in the emergence of the British Voice Association, which encompasses a wide membership of people such as otolaryngologists, speech pathologists, voice teachers and singing teachers. Yet, in spite of the high profile that voice now enjoys and despite the fact that most authors on psychogenic voice disorders recognise that there are psychological causes that need to be treated alongside voice therapy, there is little published that describes therapeutic programmes for psychogenic voice disorders.

During the years 1983–1988 we combined our skills in voice therapy and clinical psychology to treat psychogenic voice disorders which had not responded to traditional approaches. Our aim in working together initially was to understand this group of patients better and explore whether specific psychological intervention would improve the outcome. Although there is still a need for fully controlled studies and generalisations are always difficult to make from small populations, the results have been promising (Butcher et al., 1987) and this book has developed out of our collaborative work. Despite the growing awareness of team and more holistic approaches in the years since we began working together, we are not aware of any other collaborative approaches for this otherwise unresponsive population.

It has also been our impression as speech pathologists that the psychological approaches and skills being applied in treating voice disorders were limited. To assess this, in 1988 we carried out a survey of current practice and training within our profession in the UK on the treatment of psychogenic voice disorders (Elias et al., 1989). The available literature, the results of our survey and the results of our collaborative treatment all point to the importance of further training for the speech pathologist who manages patients with psychogenic voice disorders.

Our survey suggested that there were a number of uncertainties among speech pathologists working with psychogenic voice disorders. This was particularly true regarding psychological and psychiatric aspects of treatment, where the survey highlighted considerable uneasiness on the part of the clinicians. First, only 58% of voice therapists usually felt confident working with psychogenic voice disorders. Second, as many as 70% would still welcome further training in the treatment of voice disorders from a clinically involved psychologist or psychiatrist and several respondents felt that more post-qualification courses should be available than there are at present. Third, 82% of voice therapists would have liked better access to a psychologist.

The findings of the questionnaire confirmed our beliefs that there are insufficient techniques taught at undergraduate level for treatment of this group of patients. The questionnaire also revealed that during training the management of psychologically based speech and language disorders tends to be dealt with theoretically rather than through illustration with practical applications. We are firmly of the opinion that the latter should be incorporated into the training of speech pathology students.

In addition, the responses to our survey demonstrated that the speech pathologist is frequently not equipped with the skills of conducting a psychological interview and, consequently, the management of the voice disorder is restricted. Thus, apart from the treatment gap existing for the minority of patients unresponsive to speech therapy, there appears to be an overall need for more training in psychological skills and support from an appropriate specialist. This view is shared by Aronson (1990a) in the USA, who writes from his experience of American speech pathologists, and it is notable that the third edition of his text *Clinical Voice Disorders* has now been extended to include a chapter on psychologic interviewing and counselling for voice disorders. He states that 'speech pathologists need to consider their training incomplete until they have learned the basic skills of psychologic interviewing and counselling' (p.259), and he explains that these skills are essential when diagnosing voice disorders, assessing when other psychodiagnostic or psychotherapeutic help is needed and to ensure that the therapist is a more skilled clinician. We too consider that the psychological interview is an essential addition to the speech pathologist's repertoire: first in deciding the aetiology of the psychogenic voice disorder; second, as an early predictor of the patient's potential to change patterns of thinking and behaviour, which may be perpetuating the problem; and third as a means of collecting information that will suggest the appropriate treatment strategies.

Concerning the standard of counselling skills in the UK, our impression during our collaboration has been that even when these are of a high level in terms of the therapist being more than proficient in client-centred counselling techniques (Rogers, 1951, 1961), these skills alone were not always sufficient to facilitate change. Our observation was that the therapists work more effectively once they acquire a better understanding of cognitive–behavioural psychology and related treatment techniques. Therefore it is our conclusion that the speech pathologist needs to be more fully trained in the practical application of psychological treatment approaches in order to work more effectively and efficiently with psychogenic voice disorders.

Since the literature is confused about diagnosis and classification of psychogenic voice disorders, we begin this book with a review of the classification systems used, describe common characteristics of psychogenic voice disorders, consider how successful traditional voice therapy is for this population and explore the value of a more psychological approach to treatment.

Chapter 2 provides an overview of current psychological approaches that are most frequently used by speech pathologists in their treatment of a range of disorders. The bulk of the book is then devoted to describing the cognitive–behavioural model, both theoretically in Chapter 3 and then clinically in Chapters 4–6. Psychological interviewing and assessment techniques are described in Chapter 4 and the application of cognitive–behavioural treatment techniques to voice disorders in Chapter 5. In the final chapter we have added a further dimension to the book by suggesting other clinical areas where a cognitive–behavioural model could be applied in speech pathology.

The book has been written primarily for speech pathology clinicians and students. However, we expect that other professional groups such as psychologists, psychiatrists and ear, nose and throat consultants and their teams, including voice clinic personnel, will also find it of interest. Two important aims of the book are to provide speech pathologists with an introduction to cognitive–behavioural assessment techniques and to illustrate a variety of treatment strategies which can be applied when dealing with different types of problems.

This book is intended to be an introductory text only, but we hope that clinicians will also find it helpful in clarifying their own thoughts about the management of individual patients. It is not our intention that speech pathologists should use the techniques without appropriate supervision. Rather, we hope that the book will encourage further training in psychological skills and the development of working links with an interested psychologist or psychiatrist for discussion and supervision. There are many courses available at the postgraduate level for training therapists in cognitive–behavioural skills. The trained therapist may then use this book as a guide for the treatment of psychogenic voice disorders and other communication disorders when using the cognitive–behavioural approach.

It is to the speech pathologist that voice disorders are commonly referred. Although some patients may be referred to a psychologist or psychiatrist for therapy, they seem to be a minority. This may in part be due to the limited availability of such services but it is also recognised (Koufman and Blalock 1982; Carding and Horsley, 1992) that voice therapy is largely an effective intervention. A patient who has sought investigation from an otolaryngologist for a difficulty with his or her voice is likely to find referral to a voice therapist more acceptable than referral to a psychology department. The speech pathologist will have a broad knowledge base of voice dysfunction and will be able to assess the patient against that background. The underlying psychological causes of the dysphonia may become clearer as the speech pathologist works initially through direct voice therapy. Having built a rapport with the patient and acquired insight into how emotions and stresses are contributing to the dysphonia, the speech pathologist is well placed to intervene further at a psychological level. For the patient, disclosing information of an emotional kind can be less difficult once a trusting relationship has been established and, for the speech pathologist, tackling the psychological issue can be a natural extension of the voice therapy. The alternative options open to the speech pathologist are either to refer on to a psychologist or psychiatrist or to decide to restrict the scope of therapy to direct voice intervention, perhaps with some Rogerian-style counselling. Finding a psychologist or psychiatrist interested and willing to accept the patient may be difficult, particularly in the numbers that may present, but one should perhaps question whether this is the most appropriate course of management since the patient may receive interrupted care and the psychologist and psychiatrist may not have the knowledge of the normal and abnormal voice.

These seem sound reasons for suggesting that equipping the speech pathologist with psychological skills is a good investment. These skills would be accessed for many patients, not only for the more complex psychogenic dysphonics, and thus enhance the quality of intervention. For example, many voice disorders that have arisen from habitual misuse have a psychogenic dimension and therefore the speech pathologist needs to combine voice therapy with the appropriate counselling in order to resolve the underlying psychological factors.

While reading and knowledge alone will not produce a skilled cognitive–behavioural therapist, we believe that most speech pathologists who are properly supervised and supported in developing these skills, particularly through working in collaboration with an experienced therapist or psychologist, can eventually work more independently and that this will lead to a more effective and economic treatment for psychogenic voice disorders. Encouragingly, there is a growing interest within the profession in the UK in the provision for staff of formal clinical supervision in casework (Green, 1992). This is a welcome move forward and parallels the ways other professions, such as social workers and psychotherapists, are working.

In conclusion, we offer in this book a combined approach: voice therapy using a specific psychological model. Our clinical experience has shown this to be beneficial with a difficult group of voice patients. We hope that the book will be similarly helpful in the work of speech pathologists engaged with voice disorders and that they will consider the application of the model to other areas of speech pathology.

In concluding, we would like to acknowledge the invaluable contributions from Mrs Jenny Yeatman, senior speech and language therapist at The Royal London Hospital. It was with her early clinical collaboration that the ideas for this book first emerged and we are much indebted to her efforts in bringing it to publication.

We would like to thank our secretaries, Miss Debra Barker and Mrs Laura Harvey, for their patience and time in drafting this work. These acknowledgements would not be complete without our thanks to our families for their support in enabling us to maintain our domestic and working lives while writing this book.

Finally, we owe a great deal to the various advisors who read and commented on the earlier drafts and whose constructive comment helped to shape this final text. We should acknowledge in particular Dr Daniel Boone, and also Dr Arnold Aronson, whose own work and generous encouragement has inspired us.

Peter Butcher
Annie Elias
Ruth Raven
February 1993

Contents

Chapter 3

Chapter 4

Chapter 5

Chapter 6

The application of cognitive–behaviour therapy in speech and language therapy

Chapter 1
Psychological Voice Disorders

The human voice is an individual and highly developed function of the larynx. The larynx is a complicated organ consisting of a cartilaginous framework joined together by a system of muscles and ligaments. The vocal folds form the vibrating part of the larynx. As we exhale an airstream through the larynx, the vibrating vocal folds generate the sound wave producing vocal tone.

We use voice to give expression and meaning to our language. The different features of the voice combine to convey meaning and communicate our message effectively. The listener is helped to interpret the subtleties of the language through the nuances of the speaker's voice.

If a person's voice changes persistently or repeatedly, then he or she will usually detect the change and seek a medical opinion. 'A voice disorder exists when quality, pitch, loudness or flexibility differs from the voices of others of similar age, sex and cultural group' (Aronson, 1990a, p.6). Typically the voice disorder is attributed either to organic pathology, brought about through congenital disorder, inflammation, tumour, endocrine disorder, trauma or neurological disease, or to a non-organic origin. It is the role of the ear, nose and throat surgeon to make a medical diagnosis and to exclude organic disease before making a diagnosis of non-organic disorder.

There is a strong relationship between the voice and the rest of the body. Therefore the speech pathologist is concerned with posture, body use and breathing. Our voices are so much a part of our inner selves that they are affected by our thoughts, our emotions and our relationship with ourselves. Our voices are also considerably influenced by environment and relationships with other people. We cannot completely conceal how we feel; our voices communicate our emotions. If we feel liberated and vibrant our voices sound open and energetic. If we feel hurried and impatient, our voices sound quick and sharp. If we are convulsed by sobbing, our voices are broken and uncontrolled. When describing the voice of the singer and actor, Punt (1979, p.3) explains 'The vocal mechanism may be healthy and

1

undamaged, but the precision with which it responds to the subtle and intricate demands made upon it is so often affected by the state of mind and emotions of the performer'. The relationship that our voices have with ourselves and with the listener is described by Shewell (1990):

> Voice is a genuinely psychosomatic phenomenon. It not only expresses the state of the speaker's psyche (personality and feelings) and soma (body), it also has an effect on the psyche and soma of the person hearing it.

(p.15)

The term 'psychological voice disorder' implies that there is an observable voice problem and that the causative and perpetuating factors are largely psychological. The literature abounds with varying opinions about the nature of these disorders. In this chapter we shall present our own observations of psychological voice disorders and their general characteristics as described in the literature. We then look more specifically at a group of patients who do not respond to traditional speech therapy techniques and finally suggest an alternative approach to managing them.

Terminology

Voice disorders with predominant psychological features are referred to variously as 'psychogenic', 'functional', 'psychosomatic', 'hysterical' and 'non-organic'. These are defined as those conditions 'that exist in the absence of organic laryngeal pathology' (Aronson, 1990a, p.120) and as 'the product of both laryngeal and supralaryngeal shut down' (Boone and McFarlane, 1988, p.53). We found from our survey into current practice and training in the UK (Elias et al., 1989) that the term 'functional' was most commonly applied, although the four other descriptions were also in use.

The difficulty with terms such as 'functional' or 'non-organic' is that they fail to specify the underlying cause and are now less used to refer to other psychogenic disorders. Aronson describes the ambiguity of the term 'functional' when applied to voice disorders and cites Perello (1962), who found eight interpretations of 'functional voice disorder'. It is now acknowledged that the functional–organic dichotomy is too simplistic a view for voice disorders and indeed that the term 'functional' is less useful and may become increasingly redundant for classifying voice disorders (Freeman, 1991). The term 'hysterical' implies a single psychological mechanism, which may not always operate. Indeed, it was found from a study by House and Andrews (1987, p.483) that of several hundred cases in two clinics 'no more than 4–5% of those with so-called functional voice disorder could be diagnosed as true hysterical aphonia'. Aronson (1990a) explains the common error of using the terms 'hysteria' and 'conversion' interchangeably and describes the distinguishing characteristics of each. While we would not feel uncomfortable about using the term 'psychosomatic', particularly as it conveys an important connection between mind and physical symptoms, an unfortunate popular belief concerning this term is that the physical symptoms are 'all in the mind' of the patient or are imaginary rather than real. This is clearly not the case with the types of dysphonias we are discussing.

To this discussion of terminology we should add the labels, 'hyperkinetic', 'hyperfunctional' and 'habitual dysphonia'. These typically refer to vocal misuse and abuse where the dysphonia has arisen as a result of excessive tension in the vocal tract and in particular in the intrinsic laryngeal muscles. This may or may not lead to changes in the laryngeal mucosa.

Since the dysphonias being examined in this book are of psychological origin or primarily related to psychological processes, we have concluded that they are best referred to as 'psychogenic' and it is therefore this term that we will use throughout the book. Nevertheless, as the following discussion on classification will illustrate, one cannot necessarily infer from a psychogenic voice disorder the absence of physiological dysfunction or organic change.

Classification of psychogenic voice disorder

Just as there is not total agreement on the terminology used to describe psychogenic voice disorders, there is a similar confusion with their classification. Speech pathologists who are expert in the field of voice disorders show considerable variation in their classification of them. Their opinions reflect the extent to which they see psychological causes influencing voice disorders. Aronson (1990a), for example, extends his classification of psychogenic voice disorder to include vocal abuse.

The four main categories of voice disorder that Aronson includes as psychogenic are as follows:

1. *Musculoskeletal tension disorders*, which include vocal abuse, vocal nodules, contact ulcers and ventricular dysphonia.
2. *Conversion voice disorders*, which include conversion muteness and aphonia, conversion dysphonia and psychogenic adductor spastic dysphonia.
3. *Mutational falsetto* (puberphonia).
4. *Childlike speech in adults*.

Other authorities on voice, e.g. Boone and McFarlane (1988) and Greene and Mathieson (1989), largely confine their classification of psychogenic or functional voice disorders to those disorders that are non-organic and are 'a reflection of underlying psychological problems' (Greene and Mathieson, 1989, p.161). These same authors classify hyperkinetic dysphonias as quite separate from psychogenic dysphonias, although they clearly acknowledge that emotional stresses and psychogenic factors can partly cause or perpetuate the hyperkinetic dysphonia. The terms such as hyperkinetic, hyperfunctional and habitual dysphonia, which describe dysphonias that arise from mechanical misuse, seem to be synonymous with Aronson's label of musculoskeletal tension disorder, the difference being that Aronson categorises musculoskeletal tension disorders as psychogenic. Perhaps the decision as to whether a voice disorder might be termed hyperkinetic or hyperfunctional rather than psychogenic is more a question of the degree to which underlying emotional stresses contribute to the dysphonia and of the degree of influence that those stresses have in perpetuating patterns of excessive laryngeal tension. To illustrate simply, a teacher who has acquired a faulty voice production as a result of teaching during laryngitis and who may have some symptoms of tension, mainly as a result of the difficulties caused by the dysphonia, could be clearly diagnosed as suffering from vocal misuse. In contrast, in the case of another teacher, who has acquired a similar dysphonia in similar circumstances but who was coming to terms with a stressful divorce, the assessment may be that the life stresses had played a major part in triggering the dysphonia because increased muscle tension was present before the laryngitis, making the voice more vulnerable. The degree to which the dysphonia might be classed as habitual or psychogenic is likely to influence the type of treatment needed. A typically habitual or hyperkinetic dysphonia, as in the first example, is likely to respond to symptomatic voice therapy, whereas a dysphonia resulting more from emotional stresses and more easily termed psychogenic, as in the second example, is more likely to need a psychological approach. The difficulty here is in presenting an oversimplification of the facts because of the interrelationship between the hyperfunctional voice and the increased muscle tension which can be caused both by bad vocal habits and by emotional stress.

Aronson sees a strong connection between vocal abuse and psychological factors. He views personality traits and life stresses as contributory factors to these hyperkinetic or hyperfunctional dysphonias.

> Even when the nodule appears to be the sole result of abuse from singing or other strenuous vocal activity, it is often found that these were not the only factors responsible for the vocal abuse; these patients had also entered a period of their lives in which concomitant emotional stress had surfaced.
>
> *(Aronson, 1990a, p.126)*

Our own findings (Butcher et al., 1987) support Aronson's view that voice disorders resulting from excessive muscular tension may be strongly influenced by emotional factors. We therefore agree with Aronson's cardinal principle that 'the extrinsic and intrinsic laryngeal muscles are exquisitely sensitive to emotional stress and their hyper-contraction is the common denominator in virtually all psychogenic voice disorders' (Aronson, 1990a, p.212).

If we refer back to Aronson's classification of psychogenic dyspho-nia, it is the first two groups, musculoskeletal tension and conversion disorders, that most commonly present in the speech pathology clinic. Within the conversion disorders it is conversion aphonia and dys-phonia that are the most common. It is therefore worth discussing these two groups in an attempt to review what is understood about the psychogenic voice disorders that are commonly referred to the speech pathologist. We should stress at the outset that the common factor of hypercontraction of the laryngeal muscles in both groups does render classification difficult. Although these categories provide us with valu-able understanding of the factors leading to psychogenic voice disor-der, distinctions between them are not always clear cut.

Musculoskeletal tension disorders

Physical characteristics

In this group an ear, nose and throat examination will reveal the vocal folds to be normal or mildly inflamed; they may not fully adduct or they may be slightly bowed or, conversely, hyperadduct. Although, if the voice is continually produced abnormally, some structural changes may occur in the larynx, leading for example to inflammation, the for-mation of nodules and contact ulcers, such structural change is often minimal or absent. Aronson (1990a, p.121) explains, 'In general, how-ever, the extent of visible pathology is incongruously minor or absent in comparison with the severity of abnormal voice'. Part of the tension is due to retraction of the tongue and part to elevation of the larynx and hyoid bone, which can be detected manually by the clinician. The patient may experience laryngeal discomfort and feelings of 'a lump in the throat', tightness or difficulty in swallowing. The use of xeroradi-ograms has enabled the therapist to observe the muscular changes around the larynx, which are responsible for the dysphonic voice (MacCurtain, 1983). Furthermore, the use in some ear, nose and throat clinics of video stroboscopy provides a detailed view of the vocal fold movement on phonation. This investigation directly highlights the pre-cise nature of excess tension in the region of the vocal folds during speech. The description given by Boone (1977) of functional dyspho-nia shares the characteristics of musculoskeletal tension dysphonia. Boone (1977, p.58) states that a 'functionally caused dysphonia does not necessarily sound different from an organically caused one. The same subjective terms (harsh, hoarse, breathy, strident, weak, etc.) are commonly used to describe both'. Generally, musculoskeletal tension leads to dysphonia, but it can produce aphonia.

Aetiology

Most authors accept that psychogenic voice disorders reflect an emotional cause. Some authors suggest that certain personality traits are responsible for the dysphonia. Aronson (1990a, p.121) describes common factors responsible for the hypercontraction of the intrinsic and extrinsic laryngeal muscles as being 'anxiety, anger, irritability, impatience, frustration and depression'. Luchsinger and Arnold (1965) explain that states of tension arise both from exogenous sources, which are environmental factors such as work or family difficulties, and from endogenous sources which relate to the individual's personality, for example, perfectionism, compulsive attitudes, overambitious drives. The result of sustained tension without appropriate release leads to unnecessarily high muscular tonus.

Since the larynx is in a continual state of hypercontraction in this type of dysphonia, a traditional theory for onset has been poor vocal technique. However, it does not automatically follow that poor vocal technique is a necessary cause of the dysphonia and 'there is no good evidence that a job involving above-average voice use is a particular risk factor' (House and Andrews, 1987, p.484). Indeed, rather than being a cause, poor vocal technique may more commonly result from attempts to compensate for voice loss where there is already increased musculoskeletal tension.

Conversion voice disorders

Physical characteristics

Conversion aphonia and dysphonia present a similar physical picture to musculoskeletal tension disorders, although the vocal folds will typically be normal. Greene and Mathieson (1989) review the positions that the vocal folds adopt in conversion aphonia. The vocal folds may not attempt to adduct for voice or, alternatively, may be tightly adducted in a spasm of both adductor and constrictor laryngeal muscles. Such hyperadduction will include the adduction of the ventricular folds. A considerable variety of whispers may be present and excess muscular tension is a feature: 'The sharpness of the whispering indicates that the intrinsic laryngeal muscles are in a state of hypercontraction, even though the vocal folds are prevented from approximating' (Aronson,

1990a, p.131). In conversion dysphonia we see 'varying degrees and types of hoarseness, with and without a strained-harsh quality, high-pitched falsetto breaks, breathiness, intermittent whispering with moments of breathy and normal voice, and other variants too numer-ous, diverse and indescribable to mention' (Aronson, 1990a, p.134). In both aphonic and dysphonic patients there is the same excessive laryn-geal tension and common complaint of discomfort and pain in the lar-ynx as there is in the musculoskeletal tension group.

Aetiology

Traditionally, conversion disorders were labelled 'hysterical', a term originating from Hippocrates' belief that the condition was limited solely to women and was caused by a wandering womb (*hystera* being the Greek word for uterus). Characteristically in these disorders we find that motor or sensory functions are impaired (including full or partial paralysis of limbs, loss of sensations, insensitivity to pain, tunnel vision or complete blindness) without the presence of neurological impairment. The patients sometimes appear quite unperturbed by their condition and *la belle indifference* can be an important diagnostic fea-ture. Symptoms commonly appear during periods of stress and can serve the function of helping the sufferer avoid a decision, responsibili-ty, action or relationship difficulties. The symptoms may also increase attention and support from others, which may be highly desired or rewarding.

Freud was the first to use the term 'conversion disorder' to describe these conditions because he believed that the energy associated with repressed sexual and aggressive instincts became channelled or *con-verted* into physical symptoms by blocking the normal functioning of sensorimotor pathways.

> Freud considered the specific nature of the hysterical symptom to relate either to the repressed instinctual urge or to its repressing counterforce, representing them in disguised form. A hysterical convulsion might be the symbolic expression of a forbidden sexual wish, a hysterical paralysis the manifestation of self-punishment for a hidden aggressive urge.
>
> *(Davison and Neale, 1982, p.180)*

Another example of how a conversion symptom can be a symbol of unconscious conflict would be to conclude that a person suffering from conversion blindness does not wish to see something which caus-es distress and that the blindness also has value to the patient by increasing the attention and caring behaviour of others.

The Freudian view of the aetiology of hysterical conversion disorders has been more influential than any other in shaping our understanding of this condition. Aronson (1990a, p.129) follows the psychoanalytic tradition by stating that the disorders may be interpreted as serving 'the psychologic purpose of enabling the patient to avoid awareness of emotional conflict, stress, or personal failure that would be emotionally intolerable if faced directly'.

While it is clear that interpretations of aetiology can be made using psychoanalytic theory and while some of these constructs are valuable, it may not be necessary to embrace these theories wholeheartedly. Given that recent research involving studies of several hundreds of cases of non-organic voice disorder indicated that only 4–5% of these patients could be confidently diagnosed as genuine conversion or hysterical aphonia (cited by House and Andrews, 1987), it may be that only a minority of psychogenic voice disorders are truly conversion disorders in the sense described by Freud. In relation to this, although there is some support for the psychoanalytic view that suppressed expression of anger plays a part in the voice disorder (see below), there is less evidence in the more common psychogenic aphonias and dysphonias for the psychoanalytic view that these might be associated with the unconscious repression of sexual instincts. For example, although Aronson et al. (1966) noted the presence of confusion and insecurity around sexuality, poor sexual identity or poor sexual adjustment in a large number of patients within their population of 27 psychogenic dysphonics, only four – notably all young women aged between 14 and 23 years – clearly showed 'complete, bland denial of sexuality or the outright expression of fear or hatred of it' (p.123). This having been said, a psychoanalytic interpretation emphasising an unconscious conflict over sexuality or repression of sexuality when applied to the aetiology of a voice disorder, such as childlike speech in an adult, may be a valuable explanatory construct. In these cases, the childlike speech may reflect conflicts and fears associated with personal independence, responsibility and mature sexuality and speaking in a childlike way symbolises the unconscious desire to remain a child.

Since the incidence of true conversion disorder is rare, it will probably not present as a common problem to the speech pathologist. It is a fact that many speech pathologists have success in treating aphonic patients with symptomatic voice therapy, as described by Boone (1977), or through counselling. However, it should be understood that when clearly diagnosed in the context of the patient's apparent detachment, lack of concern or *la belle indifference*, the aphonia will be more intractable or difficult to treat by either speech therapy or psychological methods. Psychotherapists of all persuasions tend to be pessimistic about significantly helping individuals with hysterical conversion disorders. Thus, in offering psychological therapy to patients with psychogenic voice disorder we chose not to include those individuals who were confidently diagnosed as suffering from this condition. The reasons for this are explained more fully in Chapter 4.

Before concluding this discussion of conversion disorders, we should turn briefly to spastic or spasmodic dysphonia. The claim that this dysphonia is a symptom of neurological disorder has been made, 'because occasional cases are associated with minor neurological signs such as involuntary movements or EEG abnormalities, and [it] does not apply to the majority of non-spasmodic dysphonias' (House and Andrews, 1987 p.484). However, Aronson (1990a) suggests that the symptoms of spastic dysphonia can be either psychogenic or neurological in origin. Greene and Mathieson (1989, p.178) take a similar view when they say 'there is evidence that though this condition has both psychogenic and neurological origins it may be attributed exclusively to one or other cause: either psychological or neurological'. Whether or not spastic dysphonia is a symptom of psychogenic or neurological origin, cognitive–behaviour therapy may have a role in treatment. For even when there is a neurological cause, as Greene and Mathieson (1989, p.268) rightly state, 'Psychological disturbance, such as anxiety and depression, is only to be expected from a crippling and occupational handicap...'. As will be illustrated in various examples throughout the book, cognitive–behaviour therapy has many strategies to improve lowered self-esteem and loss of personal and social confidence, as well as to relieve symptoms of anxiety and depression.

Common aetiological features of psychogenic voice disorders

From examining the physical and aetiological factors of musculoskeletal tension disorders and conversion disorders we have illustrated that the distinctions between them are not always clear. However, the following observations are considered to be relevant to most patients with psychogenic voice disorders and these may equip the reader with a broad appreciation of the common factors.

Stress and anxiety

It is now well documented that psychogenic voice disorders usually either follow an event of acute stress or are associated with stress over a long period of time (Greene and Mathieson, 1989; Aronson, 1990a). As would be expected in individuals who are stressed, anxiety is an extremely common symptom.

Conflict over speaking out

In their study in the UK, House and Andrews (1988) found that psychogenic voice disorder frequently occurred as a response to a specific sort of stress. A significantly high proportion of patients (54%) had experienced a difficulty or event which involved conflict over speaking out, while only 16% of a comparison group had such experiences. These findings closely replicate earlier observations we made of our own clinical sample, both in features associated with the dysphonia and in frequency found in the population:

> A large number of patients had considerable difficulty expressing feelings (particularly anger or resentment) and personal views. At least eight patients had demonstrable difficulties in this area. One patient said about her anger "I have to swallow it". Another patient was afraid that if she acknowledged and/or expressed her emotion she "might go to pieces". The tendency of patients not to express feelings frequently meant that they passively accepted an unfulfilling relationship without protest.
>
> *(Butcher et al., 1987, p.85)*

Aronson (1990a, p.132) has made a similar observation when noting that a large number of patients showed 'difficulty in dealing maturely and openly with feelings of anger'.

A predominantly female condition

Our observation and that of others working in this area is that psychogenic dysphonia is mainly a condition that occurs in women. In Aronson et al.'s (1966) study, 24 out of 27 psychogenic dysphonics (89%) were female. Of the 19 patients assessed by Butcher et al. (1987), 14 were women (74%) and in the largest study of this population (House and Andrews, 1987), 61 out of 71 patients were female (86%). Greene and Mathieson (1989, p.174) stated that conversion aphonia is more common in women than men, occurring in a ratio of 7:1. In a study by Barton (1960), all 20 patients were women, and in a study by Brodnitz (1969) of 74 aphonics, 62 were women.

Features of overcommitment and helplessness

In assessing the personal circumstances of our population of female dysphonics, we also noticed that these women not only tend to take on the main burden of responsibility within the family, but at the same time are often unable to make changes in an unsatisfactory situation owing to their lack of assertiveness. Like ourselves, House and Andrews (1988, p.317) also gained the impression that 'these women have a tendency to become involved in a social network in which they were overcommitted, but relatively powerless'.

Near-normal psychological adjustment

While it would appear that specific psychological factors lead to the establishment of the voice disorder, the evidence from a survey of the literature is that, in the main, patients with psychogenic voice disorder do not suffer from high levels of psychological disturbance or a major psychiatric condition. Aronson's (1990a, p.134) observation of 27 patients was that 'despite the psychoneurotic explanation for their voice signs, few have incapacitating psychiatric disturbances. In many ways they have adjusted to their anxiety or depression'. Our own study of 19 patients (Butcher et al., 1987) supports this view (only two patients – one diagnosed as suffering from a personality disorder, the other from conversion hysteria – were considered too disturbed psychologically to be offered treatment, while the other 17 were considered to be only mildly disturbed). Similarly, in their study of 71 patients, House and Andrews (1987, p.487) also found that the majority 'had insufficient symptoms to warrant any psychiatric diagnosis'. Taken as a whole, these findings indicate that while their psychological problems are above average, these patients are not seriously disturbed psychologically.

To this picture of psychological adjustment must be added the fact that clinical observations support the view that loss or impairment of voice, whatever its origin, can be a distressing experience for many patients and that experience, in itself, exacerbates the condition: 'the patient's frustration and anger elevate musculoskeletal tension, and whatever primary organic or psychogenic voice disorder existed up to that point is worsened to an even greater degree of severity' (Aronson, 1990a, p.140). Furthermore, in terms of a learning dimension, the primary voice disorder can become habitual, as illustrated by Boone (1977, p.61): 'he talks today with no voice because that is the way he talked yesterday'.

Psychogenic voice disorders unresponsive to speech and language therapy

Whilst it is reported that the majority of patients with psychogenic voice disorders respond well to a course of speech therapy, some 5–10% do not show improvement (Brodnitz, 1969; Koufman and Blalock, 1982) and these patients continue with persistent or recurrent symptoms. The speech pathologist is advised during training and in the literature to refer these patients on to a psychologist or psychiatrist. However, little is reported either on the collaboration between speech therapy and psychology/psychiatry or on the outcome of this type of intervention for this minority group. Hayward and Simmons (1982) described the need for such collaboration. Their work emphasised the high levels of tension and anxiety in the patient with dysphonia and their main focus was to set about treating this behaviourally in joint relaxation groups.

A study of patient characteristics and psychological treatment

In 1983 (Butcher and Elias, 1983) we reported on an initial joint speech therapy/psychology assessment and intervention with psychogenic voice disorder patients who had not responded to conventional speech therapy alone. In 1987 (Butcher et al., 1987) we were able to report more fully on our findings. Throughout the period of our investigation we aimed to explore the psychosocial characteristics of patients who had previously been unresponsive to speech therapy and to assess the effect of employing a specific psychological approach in their management. The suggestion of developing more effective treatment strategies for the chronic or relapsing sufferer has since been made by House and Andrews (1987), who are also of the opinion that a psychologically based treatment would be both acceptable and valuable to many of these patients. In our study we chose to offer a joint assessment and intervention employing a cognitive–behaviour approach as described, for example, by Kanfer and Goldstein (1982), Bradley and Thompson (1985) and Dryden and Golden (1986). This assessment and treatment format will be more fully explained in Chapters 3, 4 and 5. The results of treatment will be described later in this chapter, but first we will concentrate on the characteristics of the population.

In all we assessed 19 patients who had not improved with standard speech therapy. Following psychological assessment 15 were considered suitable for cognitive–behaviour therapy and 12 took up the offer of treatment, 11 of whom were female. Those who were not considered suitable and were not offered treatment consisted of a patient assessed to have a severe personality disorder, a patient suffering from a hysterical conversion disorder with marked symptoms of denial or *la belle indifférence*, a patient with spastic dysphonia, and a patient with intractable ongoing life stresses. In all these cases it was felt that they were unlikely to benefit from psychological treatment.

Results of psychological assessment

The study suggested that this population showed a number of commonly occurring characteristics. Most notable was the presence of anxiety and tension, family and interpersonal relationship difficulties (often in association with inhibition around expressing feelings or views), what we called 'the burden of responsibility' and the experience of a variety of life stresses.

Anxiety and tension

The most common psychological/behavioural factor was excessive anxiety and muscular tension. This was a feature in all but one of the 19 cases. We have assumed that the continuing presence of anxiety and muscular tension is the main reason why members of this population do not overcome their voice problems. The following sections describe the common causes of anxiety in this population.

Family or interpersonal relationship difficulties

Family and/or interpersonal relationship difficulties were the most common presenting problem and were a dominant feature in 14 cases. Seven patients described a poor marriage, or experienced marital conflicts; they communicated poorly and shared very little with their partners. Five other patients had a difficult or disturbed relationship with their only child, or with their children. In three of these patients we found a disturbed mother/child relationship over issues of control and limits with a daughter. An outstanding feature in the five cases was the considerable immaturity of the child or children, most of whom were in their teens or twenties. The parent usually had little independence, had a fragile identity and was highly controlled or dominated by the child.

As cited earlier, at least eight patients were judged to have a major difficulty in expressing feelings of anger or resentment and personal views. This personality characteristic often caused them to have to accept passively various relationship conflicts without a means of protest.

The burden of responsibility

Many of the patients had taken the onus of responsibility in their family or marriage, but staggered under the burden. In some cases, they felt they were married to passive or uncooperative partners who took little or no responsibility for the home or for such things as disciplining the children. Four patients were caught in a stressful relationship with an elderly, dependent mother. The patients had been left with, or had taken on, the main responsibility for looking after their parents. They tended to have little or no support in doing this and, even when support was available, they felt that they had to take the main responsibility for care.

Other life stresses

Along with, or in addition to, the features described above we identified an array of other stresses in this population. The most common
was working in a stressful environment or working long hours in a job,
as well as having to be a housewife and mother. For many of these
patients their loss of voice increased the stresses at work because they
were no longer able to perform their duties adequately. Other stresses
were associated with having to adjust to major life events, examples
being a family feud, isolation from a familiar environment and friends,
and bereavement.

The relationship between life events or difficulties preceding the
onset of psychogenic dysphonia has since been reported by House and
Andrews (1988). Our observations above are supported by their study,
which suggests that the presenting dysphonia is associated with the
experience of difficult life events at some time preceding the onset of
dysphonia.

A model of psychogenic voice disorder

In summary, our findings were that those voice patients who are unresponsive to speech therapy are commonly suffering from a condition of
protracted anxiety; many have taken on excessive responsibilities or are
subject to notable life stresses and are frequently embroiled in family
and interpersonal relationship difficulties, with a high proportion having difficulties in assertiveness and the expression of negative feelings.
This led us to conclude that, with these conditions present and particularly when an individual is involved in interpersonal conflicts wherein
they are unable to express themselves or have to 'choke back' their
feelings, such a person will be susceptible to voice loss and more difficult to treat by conventional means.

When discussing the aetiology for conversion voice disorders earlier
in this chapter, we noted that the psychoanalytic theory has provided
the main explanation for this group of disorders. This theory suggests
that voice disorder occurs as a defence against the revelation of unacceptable feelings or instincts and that the instinctual energy is convert-
ed into physical symptoms, which, in fact, symbolise the hidden or
underlying nature of the unconscious conflict. From our observations,
however, we have concluded that the loss of voice need not be an
unconscious or symbolic avoidance of expression in the psychodynam-
ic sense, but simply an involuntary difficulty connected with the high
levels of anxiety and stress which are usually associated with problematic interpersonal relationships and inhibition surrounding verbal
expression. The inhibition or conflict does not have to be unconscious
and the voice loss need not be 'symbolic'. Essentially, stressful life

events, interpersonal conflicts and difficulty over expressing feelings produce musculoskeletal tension which inhibits voice production. Although the involuntary muscular tension may reflect a fear of, or conflict over, the expression of feelings, this and other external stresses are enough to explain the symptoms without recourse to other hypothetical psychoanalytic constructs. In support of this view, we mentioned earlier that when House and Andrews (1988) reported their study of life events and difficulties preceding the onset of functional dysphonia, they included a specific feature of 'conflict over speaking out' and found that this was highly correlated with psychogenic voice loss. They too hypothesised that the voice disorder arises from muscle tension, restricted to the larynx, in response to conflict over speaking out.

In further support of this view it should be noted that many of our findings had also been anticipated by Aronson et al. (1966) in the study mentioned earlier of 27 patients diagnosed with functional voice disorder. Using both psychiatric assessment and the Minnesota Multiphasic Personality Inventory, they revealed the following. First, acute and chronic situational conflicts were found in the overwhelming majority of patients. Second, a high number, 18, were observed to be markedly immature, with histories of long dependence, and 16 had made a neurotic adjustment to life. Nevertheless, no serious psychopathology warranting immediate psychiatric help was found in any patient in this study. Third, the authors found that 'one of the most striking features about the patients of this group was their inability to deal maturely with feelings of anger' (p.119).

At the beginning of the chapter we expressed a preference for the term 'psychogenic' when discussing functional dysphonias. Taken as a whole, the above research offers important evidence for a link between dysphonia and social, interpersonal and psychological stress, especially when the latter is associated with difficulty in expressing feelings or views, and strengthens the case for functional dysphonia to be seen as a psychologically based syndrome.

Common management of psychogenic voice disorders

Referral to speech pathology

Once the ear, nose and throat surgeon has assessed the health and function of the vocal folds, it is customary to make a referral to the speech pathologist. There is agreement that this is the correct first step in the management of the patient with a psychogenic voice disorder.

In a survey which set out to assess the attitudes and practices of speech pathologists in the UK (Elias et al., 1989), we found that the majority of speech pathologists (75%) always treated psychogenic dysphonia or aphonia when patients were referred to them and a small minority (2.5%) opted never to treat these patients, the remainder selecting whether or not to treat. In this survey about three-quarters of the therapists indicated that these patients 'usually' improved. The opinion of the remaining therapists was equally divided between those who 'always' saw improvement and those who 'sometimes' did.

The therapist's skills and techniques

During training the speech pathologist becomes equipped to understand the mechanics of voice production, to recognise different qualities and to attribute these to the appropriate type of vocal dysfunction. The therapist uses a range of therapeutic techniques in order to modify vocal dysfunction and to re-establish normal voice production. Since various authors (for example, Perkins, 1957; Murphy, 1964; Greene, 1972; Freeman, 1986; Aronson, 1990a) have recognised that the psychological causes of the voice disorder need to be treated simultaneously during voice therapy, the therapist is usually encouraged to take a holistic approach to the management of the patient.

The voice interview

The ability to gather appropriate information, through skill of interviewing, is a central part of the speech pathologist's working method. Here the speech pathologist understands the importance of case history information and is attentive to the environmental and personal factors surrounding the onset and duration of the voice disorder. There are many texts which offer good advice for interviewing the patient with a voice disorder, for example: Darley and Spriestersbach (1963), Darley (1964), Boone (1977), Freeman (1986), Greene and Mathieson (1989) and Aronson (1990a).

The general advice focuses on two main areas: first, close observation of the patient's posture and behaviour in the clinic with particular attention to signs of tension; second, these observations should be combined with sensitive, well planned questioning to help reveal a full medical and voice history as well as information regarding the personal and environmental influences surrounding the onset and duration of the voice disorder.

The advice extended to speech pathologists does not specifically describe a psychological model of interviewing. The therapist may glean a rich array of information, but the scope and usefulness of the psychological history may be limited and the therapist may be restricted in the interpretations of the facts that have been gathered. The therapist may choose to ignore the psychological history altogether. Recently Aronson (1990b) has suggested that, because the speech pathologist is unpractised and unprepared in eliciting information from the patient about psychological stress and problems, the real causes behind the dysphonia go undetected. This leaves both the therapist and the patient disadvantaged in resolving the voice disorder.

Treatment techniques

There are various manuals and textbooks which advocate techniques that the speech pathologist can employ when treating a patient with a psychogenic voice disorder. For example: Boone (1977), Freeman (1986), Martin (1987), Greene and Mathieson (1989), Aronson (1990a), Boone (1991), Martin and Darnley (1992).

Most authors acknowledge that restoring normal voice is not the sole objective of therapy. Instead, the speech pathologist should help the patient to gain insight into the factors precipitating and prolonging the voice disorder and enable the patient to make some adjustments so that he or she can either alleviate the cause of the problem or modify his or her response to it. The implication is that, once the underlying cause of the problem is resolved, the voice will be improved. According to Freeman (1986):

> The clinician's first goal, then, is to help the patient to identify and work through the underlying problem, rather than concentrate therapy on the mechanisms of the voice disorder; the voice disorder is secondary to this.

(p.193)

In our UK survey (Elias et al., 1989), we undertook to discover what techniques the speech pathologist was taught for managing psychogenic voice disorders and what was being used in practice. The results, illustrated in Table 1.1, suggest that the treatment techniques used are mainly relaxation, voice exercises and counselling with a range of other, largely psychological techniques each employed by a minority of speech pathologists.

The survey also found that postqualification courses on psychogenic voice disorders, or on techniques useful for treating them, had been attended by 37% of speech pathologists. It is likely that many of these courses imparted psychological techniques, since Table 1.1 shows that, while relaxation and voice exercises were predominantly taught in pre-qualification courses, there was a trend for psychological techniques to have been learnt subsequently. In addition, the finding from the questionnaire, that counselling was much more freely advocated than taught, corresponded with comments from a number of therapists, who stated that it was important but not as extensively taught as needed. Fawcus (1986, p.11) has suggested that, rather than necessarily

Table 1.1 Treatment techniques used

	Used in practice		Encountered on initial educationcourses	
	Learnt in initial course	Learnt since initial course	Advocated	Taught
Relaxation	219	54	241	223
Voice exercises	201	84	224	191
Counselling	126	128	209	104
Behaviour therapy	39	45	44	28
Personal construct therapy	24	49	37	15
Psychotherapy	13	24	*	*
Hypnosis	4	41	20	2
Diaphragmatic breathing	*	*	213	189

* Not asked in questionnaire.

referring on for psychiatric treatment, we need first to be sure that 'careful management in terms of environmental modification, counselling and vocal remediation by the therapist is not the more appropriate course of action'. The literature, personal experience, and the results of this survey confirm that voice therapy is effective for the majority of patients with a psychogenic voice disorder. Unfortunately, there is little in the literature or from our survey that adequately describes the 'counselling' skills that are taught to, and needed by, the speech pathologist. It is assumed, however, that these skills refer largely to a Rogerian client-centred style of counselling (Rogers, 1951), in which the therapist is essentially an attentive, sympathetic and non-judgemental listener. This model of counselling will be discussed more fully in Chapter 2 but appears to be much as Greene (1972) intended when she said:

> The most important aspect of treatment is the establishment of a sympathetic and understanding relationship with the patient, who must feel able to talk freely to someone who understands how she feels. Discussion with an impartial listener gives the support a patient craves until a degree of security and confidence returns.

(p.184)

Whilst the speech pathologist may be well placed to tackle the management of the patient with a psychogenic voice disorder, there is some unease, first, that the UK survey suggests that there is a question as to the general standard of counselling skills acquired in training and, second, that, since some patients present with quite complex psychological problems, counselling skills alone may not be sufficient to treat this group. There is nothing in the texts for speech pathologists or in the results of the UK survey that gives us confidence to believe that the therapist's counselling skills are at an adequate level of sophistication for this minority of patients. In support of this, our clinical experience is that this patient group is unresponsive to traditional methods of speech therapy (Butcher and Elias, 1983; Butcher et al., 1987).

Summarising the need for psychological skills

For the reasons stated above, a speech pathologist would not be fully equipped to work with all patients who have a psychogenic voice disorder. This can be summarised as follows:

1. A minority of patients (5–10%) do not show improvement from traditional methods of voice therapy.
2. A proportion of these patients present with complex psychological problems which will not be resolved by a Rogerian client-centred style of counselling.
3. The speech pathologist is not sufficiently trained in the use of psychological constructs and in conducting a psychological interview, both of which are necessary skills in order to make full use of the case history information.
4. Overall, the extent of the speech pathologist's psychological training and skills is not sufficient to deal with this minority group of patients.

House and Andrews (1987) discuss the 5–10% of patients who continue with persistent or recurrent symptoms despite speech therapy:

> These patients do not have a good reputation for compliance with speech therapy and a clearer picture of the psychosocial characteristics of patients with functional dysphonia might lead to the development of more effective treatment strategies for the chronic or relapsing sufferer.
>
> *(p.489)*

The study described earlier of patients who had not responded to traditional speech therapy (Butcher et al., 1987) suggested that using a more sophisticated or comprehensive psychological approach can be of benefit for some patients in this population. The results of offering cognitive–behaviour therapy are depicted in Table 1.2, which illustrates that, of the 12 patients seen for joint cognitive–behaviour therapy, 50% showed an improvement in voice. Although we have pointed out a number of drawbacks in our study, such as the emphasis on clinical impression rather than on more objective or reliable forms of data collection, it was encouraging that observable changes had occurred in a group that was apparently untreatable and had failed to respond previously to traditional speech therapy.

This suggests that there were key elements in our therapy programme that met a need. These were probably the skills and specific treatment offered by the clinical psychologist and the joint working

Table 1.2 Details of 19 patients with psychogenic voice disorders unresponsive to standard speech therapy and those offered joint cognitive–behaviour therapy

	Male			Female	
	Aphonia	Dysphonia	Spastic dysphonia	Aphonia	Dysphonia
Failed speech therapy	1	3	1	4	10
Offered joint therapy	0	2	0	3	9
Entered joint therapy	–	1	–	2	9
Responded to joint therapy	–	0	–	2	4

approach. We noted from our initial work (Butcher and Elias, 1983) that the joint sessions provide an ideal way for the speech pathologist to observe and assimilate the psychological skills which apparently seem necessary for working more successfully with this type of patient. The speech pathologists found that the joint work had influenced their subsequent therapy and led to adjustments in the individual treatment they offered to other dysphonic patients. This arose partly because the relationship between the causes of psychological disturbance and the associated voice disorder became more apparent after participating in the joint sessions, and partly because the speech pathologist could generalise on the treatment approaches used during the initial study.

This chapter has illustrated how the existing classification systems for psychogenic voice disorders can be confusing. The cognitive–behavioural model of interviewing and determining the precipitating factors does offer an alternative approach for the speech pathologist and psychologist. This model is less concerned with a medical or psychoanalytical classification and more concerned with identifying the precipitating causes of the voice disorder that may be specific or unique to the individual case. In the following chapters we describe the model and the method of working in some detail and hopefully provide others who work with voice disorders an opportunity to consider its value.

Summary

The larynx is a highly complex organ sensitive to emotional changes in the individual. It is affected by thoughts and feelings, our relationship with others and with our environment. In this way, the human voice acts rather like an 'emotional barometer'.

Traditionally, vocal dysfunction is attributed to organic or non-organic causes. The term 'psychological voice disorder' implies that there is an observable voice problem and that the causative and perpetuating factors are largely psychological. Laryngeal pathology is either absent or disproportionate to the audible features of the dysphonia and the organic–non-organic dichotomy is considered too simplistic. The labels used to describe 'psychological voice disorders' are many and there is confusion over terminology and classification.

The term 'functional' is used most commonly in the literature and by clinicians but it fails to specify the underlying cause of the voice disorder and it is open to so many different interpretations that render it both confusing and less meaningful.

Within the literature, voice specialists vary in their classification of psychogenic or functional voice disorders. Their opinions reflect the extent to which they view psychological causes as influencing the voice disorder. These different classifications of 'psychological voice disorders' influence the subsequent approach to therapy, which may be more or less based on symptom modification.

We agree with Aronson's (1990a) view that voice disorders resulting from excessive muscular tension may be strongly influenced by emotional factors and that these are therefore best classified as psychological or psychogenic voice disorders. We believe that the decision as to whether or not a voice disorder might be termed hyperkinetic or hyperfunctional rather than psychogenic is more a question of the degree that the underlying emotional stresses have in contributing to the dysphonia and the degree of influence those stresses have in perpetuating patterns of excessive laryngeal tension. This decision has important implications for the choice of treatment approach adopted.

Musculoskeletal tension disorders, described by Aronson (1990a), include vocal abuse, vocal nodules, contact ulcers and ventricular dysphonia. The vocal folds are found to be normal or mildly inflamed. The patient may commonly experience laryngeal discomfort and tightness and feelings of a 'lump in the throat'. In terms of aetiology, some authors suggest that anxiety, anger and depression are some of the psychological responses which may produce excessive laryngeal tension in certain individuals. The result of sustained tension without appropriate release leads to unnecessary high muscular tonus. Conversion aphonia and dysphonia present a similar picture to that of musculoskeletal tension disorders, although the vocal folds will typically be normal. Conversion disorders, traditionally labelled 'hysterical', characteristically present with motor or sensory dysfunction in the absence of neurological signs. The incidence of conversion disorder is rare and, unless the voice returns almost immediately with voice therapy, the aphonia is usually difficult to treat with either speech pathology or psychological methods.

Psychoanalytic theory has provided the main explanation for the cause of conversion disorders and Freud interpreted a conversion symptom as a symbol of unconscious conflict relating to either repression or sexual or aggressive instincts. Since the literature suggests that only a minority of psychogenic voice disorders are 'pure' conversion disorders as described by Freud, this explanation does not provide an aetiology for the majority of psychogenic voice disorders. However, there is some evidence for the psychoanalytic view that suppressed expression of anger often plays a part in psychogenic voice disorder.

Although the distinctions between musculoskeletal tension disorder and conversion are not always clear cut, there appear to be common features relevant to both: the condition is more usual among women and, while psychopathology is low, individuals describe high levels of anxiety and life stress as well as interpersonal conflicts, difficulty expressing views, a tendency to shoulder family burdens and feelings of helplessness. For the majority of cases it appears that a psychoanalytic explanation of unconscious conflict or 'symbolic' voice loss is not appropriate. Rather, stressful life events, interpersonal conflicts and inhibition in expressing feelings produce musculoskeletal tension which inhibits voice production. Taken as a whole, this suggests that the term 'psychogenic' best describes these voice disorders and provides more evidence for functional dysphonia to be seen as a psychologically based syndrome.

A survey carried out by Elias et al. (1989) confirmed that, currently, speech pathologists in the UK are not sufficiently trained in conducting a psychological interview and in the use of psychological techniques, both of which are necessary skills if the speech pathologist is to make full use of the case history information.

The survey confirmed the need to extend the speech pathologist's psychological training and skills in order that he or she can deal competently with psychogenic dysphonia. One way these skills can be taught is through collaborative work with a psychologist. In particular we suggest that cognitive–behaviour therapy can offer the speech pathologist a valuable means of assessment and treatment.

Chapter 2
Current Psychological Approaches used in Speech Pathology

The primary theme of this book is the use of cognitive–behaviour therapy in treating psychogenic voice disorders. However, this treatment approach needs to be put into context. First of all, there are many other psychotherapeutic theories and methods which have influenced the speech pathologist. Second, psychological approaches can have relevance not only in voice treatment but in treating the whole range of communication disorders. Thus in this chapter we will explore and evaluate the level of training in psychological skills and the place in speech pathology, generally, of psychological treatments other than cognitive–behaviour therapy. In Chapter 6 we will pick up the theme of the wider application of cognitive–behaviour therapy in speech and language dysfunction.

In reviewing the speech pathologist's current level of skill in psychological treatments and trends for commonly adopted approaches, data can be drawn from the training establishments and from the Counselling Special Interest Group within the UK. Although the data are restricted to a UK perspective, our impression is that they provide a reflection of the international picture.

Psychological skills acquired during training

As the importance of counselling has become more widely recognised within the work place, in health, education and social services, so there have been changes in the undergraduate syllabus of speech pathologists to reflect this need for more skills. This is certainly the case in the UK, where there is recognition that interpersonal, counselling or psychologically based skills need to be taught to the undergraduate. However, whilst training in these areas is seen as an essential prerequisite if the new graduate is to cope competently with clients, a survey of all the training courses carried out by Shewell (1992) reveals that there is considerable variability in the teaching of these counselling skills. Shewell's data show that there are notable variations in three areas involving the amount of time devoted to teaching psychological methods, the content of course work and the teaching methods employed. Time allocation to teaching psychological skills ranges from as little as 10 hours during one four-year course to eight times this amount on another course. The course content is usually no more than the teaching of communication and interpersonal skills and basic counselling, but some courses offer an optional advanced counselling module. The teaching methodology in this area is both experiential and knowledge based and the course content suggests that students are taught some counselling skills and client-centred counselling, as described later in this chapter. Even where advanced training in counselling is an option, the training establishments recognise that undergraduates are taught only an introduction to counselling and on graduation are not equipped as fully competent counsellors. The main consistent findings of the survey are a general agreement that counselling skills should be taught throughout the course, that more time needs to be devoted to this area, that there ought to be a recommended course syllabus and that the course content should be progressive with advanced counselling skills being taught as an option for both undergraduates and postgraduates.

As reported in both the Preface and Chapter 1, our own survey of graduate speech pathologists (Elias et al., 1989), found that counselling was not taught as extensively during training as therapists felt it should have been. The results of Shewell's more recent UK survey of teaching practices suggest that this aspect of training still needs a great deal of development and standardisation.

Psychotherapeutic skills acquired after training

The existence of the Special Interest Group in Counselling for speech pathologists in the UK reflects the growing interest in psychotherapeutic techniques. The group was formed in 1987 and, although it has a membership of well over 100 speech pathologists, this is no doubt restricted by geographical constraints since the group meets in London. Nevertheless, the group provides a significant sample of therapists interested and involved in counselling or psychotherapy and gives some indication of the range of psychological approaches used within the profession.

In 1990 the Special Interest Group surveyed its membership to examine the extent of their training and skills (Green, 1990). The returns, from 132 speech pathologists, provide a valuable overview of the various psychological theories that influence these practising clinicians. Participants were asked to describe the psychological approaches which influence their therapy. The predominant influence on therapeutic orientation (75%) was Rogerian or client-centred counselling techniques, with personal construct therapy (influencing 60%) a close second. A wide variety (26) of theoretical approaches made up the remaining, minority, influence on therapeutic orientation. Although behaviour therapy was cited by 30 speech pathologists (23%), cognitive therapy was noted as an influence by a small minority and only one speech pathologist mentioned the influence of cognitive–behaviour therapy. As can be seen from these results, the theoretical influences were not mutually exclusive and many speech pathologists are now choosing to develop their personal eclectic therapeutic styles by integrating various psychological approaches.

The predominant influences and trends

Counselling, client-centred therapy and personal construct therapy are currently most influential in the UK and these will be reviewed in more detail in this chapter. Counselling and client-centred therapy are usually classified as humanistic, existential or phenomenological, while personal construct therapy is predominantly cognitive in its orientation. However, what is missing from these classifications is a description of the behaviour-therapy strategies which have influenced speech pathologists and which speech pathologists have often employed in treatment. Thus, we will make an attempt to fill this gap by briefly describing the way in which behavioural principles have been used in speech pathology. Following this, we will describe anxiety control training, a predominantly behavioural treatment employing elements of systematic desensitisation (Wolpe, 1969), covert conditioning (Kanfer, 1982) and cognitive therapy. We have chosen anxiety control training to conclude the chapter because it is a popular, widely used approach among speech pathologists and illustrates an important trend toward developing a comprehensive treatment package for a specific need. In reviewing the above approaches our intention is to illustrate the main psychological models and methods which speech pathologists have turned to in an attempt to be more successful therapists. The chapters which follow demonstrate not only that these approaches are compatible with cognitive–behaviour therapy, but also that the latter is a model and approach which integrates humanistic, cognitive and behaviour therapy, as well as particular treatment packages (or what can often be more piecemeal, one-dimensional therapeutic efforts) into a single therapeutic format applicable to a wide variety of problems within the field of speech pathology.

The role of counselling

The term counselling has a wide definition: it can refer simply to the giving of general advice or, at the other end of the spectrum, to a much more skilled level of therapeutic involvement on the part of the practitioner. It is the skilled level of therapeutic involvement which is of greatest relevance in speech pathology. Gravell and France (1991) put it succinctly:

> It is known that there are considerable benefits from encouraging the patient to talk. The opportunity to speak to a receptive, professionally trained listener is known to be therapeutic and frequently the patient feels an improvement in his symptoms or an alleviation of distress following such an interview.

> *(p.284)*

In this context Brumfitt (1986) has written an excellent practical guide to counselling and has emphasised the skills that are necessary in order to be an effective counsellor. For example, the better knowledge we have of our selves, the more we are able to be empathic and non-judgemental as counsellors. In the field of speech pathology, Brumfitt also draws particular attention to the needs of people suffering from communication disorders, not only their need for empathy or recognition of how they feel, but also an opportunity to find a means of coming to terms with their condition. However, only when the speech pathologist is a trained counsellor can these needs be adequately met. Unfortunately, as was shown earlier, despite the increasing profile of counselling within this profession and the rising interest shown by the training establishments, speech pathologists who wish to develop these skills in the main have to seek out training for themselves at a postgraduate level.

Client- or person-centred therapy

The development in the 1940s by Carl Rogers (1902–1987) of what was to become client- or person-centred therapy was to have enormous influence on counselling and psychotherapy. Offering a much simpler account of psychological disorder and its treatment than psychoanalysis, Rogers's basic assumptions and approach have been clearly summarised by Davison and Neale (1982) as follows. First of all the therapist needs to adopt a phenomenological point of view:

> People can be understood only from the vantage point of their own perceptions and feelings. It is the way people construe events rather than the events themselves that the investigator must attend to, for the person's phenomenological world is the major determinant of behaviour and makes him or her unique.

> *(p.572)*

Second, healthy people are aware of their behaviour. Third, people are naturally good or effective but become disturbed or ineffective through faulty learning. Fourth, an individual does not respond passively to environmental or inner stimulus, but is self-directive. Fifth, the therapist should simply create conditions which will facilitate the individual's ability to make independent decisions.

It can be seen from the above that Rogers believed that people have enormous potential to understand themselves and to resolve their own problems and are capable of self-directive growth within a non-directive or uncoercive therapeutic relationship. Also, in contrast to the psychoanalytic approach, he argued how it is necessary to explore the individual's subjective awareness of here-and-now thoughts and feelings rather than attempt to analyse unconscious processes by exploring past events. In this way individuals' perceptions of themselves and their worries are then discussed and talked through with the therapist, who facilitates the drawing of realistic conclusions about their lives and themselves. As will also be shown in later chapters, this emphasis is also central to cognitive and cognitive–behaviour therapies.

As Rogers's concept of therapy evolved (from describing it as non-directive to client- or person-centred therapy), he began to place most emphasis on the attitude and personal characteristics of the therapist and the qualities of the client–therapist relationship as the prime determinants of outcome in the therapeutic process. Through being genuine, showing empathy and acceptance and caring in the form of 'unconditional positive regard' (or being non-judgemental) and through recognition and focus on the clarification of feelings, the therapist provides a client with an environment in which he or she can safely become less defensive and more open to meaningful self-exploration. The therapist's role is then to help the client clarify his or her thoughts and feelings by reflecting back, rephrasing or summarising the statements which the client has just made. This reflection should mirror the essence of what the individual is trying to express, ideally bringing out feelings which are only hinted at or half expressed. The emphasis on the 'mirroring of feelings back to the client' and the avoidance of interpretation is intended to encourage the individual to speak more openly and honestly and thereby gradually remove the emotional conflict inhibiting 'self-actualisation'. Rogers found that if this is done consistently, positive self changes occur and that this alone is mainly responsible for altering behaviour and helping the individual become his or her 'true self'.

The goals of therapy and the changes in people who enter therapy were described by Rogers (1961) as: developing an openness to experience; recognising that they have an internal source of evaluation; finding the ability to trust in themselves; and discovering a willingness to continue growing.

First of all I would say that in this process the individual becomes more open to his experience. This is a phrase which has come to have a great deal of meaning to me. It is the opposite of defensiveness ... He also becomes more aware of reality as it exists outside of himself, instead of perceiving it in preconceived categories. He sees that not all trees are green, not all men are stern fathers, not all women are rejecting, not all failure experiences prove that he is no good, and the like. He is able to take in the evidence in a new situation, *as it is*, rather than distorting to fit a pattern which he already holds. As you might expect, this increasing ability to be open to experience makes him far more realistic in dealing with new people, new situations, new problems. It means that his beliefs are not rigid, that he can tolerate ambiguity.

(p.115)

Although the terms that Rogers uses to convey the aims of therapy are different from those employed by most cognitive–behaviour therapists, later chapters will illustrate how central to both schools of thought is the focus on helping individuals to change tendencies to hold innacurate beliefs and to achieve a more realistic evaluation of themselves and their world.

Evaluation

Rogerian therapy is a humanistic, practical, relatively simple, clearly defined approach which continues to be one of the most common forms of psychotherapy used with individuals and groups. It can be used with a wide variety of emotional conditions, especially for counselling at times of stress or in crisis intervention. Its influence in counselling is enormous and many other therapy systems have their foundations in this approach. Furthermore, its simplicity makes it an approach in which the novice therapist quickly and rightly gains confidence. 'For a person with limited background in counselling psychology, personality dynamics and psychopathology, the approach offers assurance that prospective clients will not be psychologically harmed' (Corey, 1991, p.215). On the negative side, however, person-centred counselling has been shown to work well only with less severe psychological problems and, while it may not actively harm patients, empathy, genuineness and unconditional positive regard may not provide sufficient help. This has certainly been our experience in treating a number of psychogenic dysphonic patients. At the same time, we also feel that client-centred therapy is not only a valid treatment approach but is general enough for use in many different areas of speech pathology where 'counselling' skills are needed to help individuals and carers come to terms with lost or altered communication (Purser, 1982). However, one possible, additional disadvantage of using person-centred therapy alone is that, while it can be effective in brief interventions, a positive outcome may require more treatment sessions than is typically the case when cognitive–behaviour therapy is used.

Personal construct psychology

The development of personal construct theory by George Kelly (1905–1966) offers another phenomenological approach but, in comparison to client-centred therapy, it explores in much more depth the way in which the individual forms concepts or 'personal constructs' about the self and the world. In Kelly's terms a 'personal construct' refers to the individual way a person interprets, makes sense of, or attaches meaning to aspects of his or her world and him or her self. Kelly suggested that we are continually construing the world in terms of 'distinctions', forming the constructs which discriminate between two poles or contrasts.

> The importance of a personal construct is that it determines what and how a person will perceive, remember, learn, think, and act with respect to the class of elements that are encompassed by the construct. If he has the construct that all snakes are dangerous, he will try to avoid them. A construct may be thought of as a working hypothesis which is validated or invalidated by the test of experience.
>
> *(Nordby and Hall, 1974, p.104)*

In other words, Kelly emphasised how we all make predictions based upon past experience and carry out experiments to see whether these predictions are correct. Thus, central to Kelly's theory of human behaviour is the simile that each individual acts like a scientist who predicts and then tests out his or her predictions. If the test or tests show the theory is invalid, a new theory or construct is formed and tested. In this way, the individual's construct system incorporates new constructs and expands. Problems occur, however, when the person has difficulty in finding a new, accurate, realistic or appropriate explanatory construct for the events or experiences he or she encounters. For example, Kelly (1955, p.500) stated that the cause of anxiety is a 'failure to produce a construction that appears wholly applicable to the events of which one is aware'.

Kelly also highlighted how there are many different types of constructs. *High level* constructs are always verbal and *low level* constructs are usually non-verbal. Among the non-verbal constructs are those which are *preverbal*. These develop before speech and are usually related to basic needs, for example, needs for love, warmth, physical contact and feeding. *Core* and *peripheral* constructs are vital to the individual's identity and self-definition. Core role constructs relate to oneself and one's social interactions. Peripheral constructs can be changed or altered more easily with less effect on the individual. *Permeable* and *impermeable* constructs are those which either allow or disallow new elements. *Tight* constructs are those where the same predictions are made repeatedly and where behaviour is habitual and rigid. We need tight constructs for some situations but they can be limiting in others. *Loose* constructs are 'sketchier', more flexible and 'permit predictions to vary, depending on the situation and other factors' (Nordby and Hall, 1974, p. 106).

An important concept which Kelly introduced, and which is related to tight and loose constructs and personal change, was the creativity cycle. Kelly highlighted how, in the complexity of life, adaptive functioning is possible only if we loosen or widen constructs which are too constricting or limiting. Once the construct is loosened and becomes more open, it will be necessary to build in some constraints or to tighten the construct so that there are boundaries, guidelines, exceptions and so on for the new way of thinking and acting. New information or challenges to this construct, or to other constructs, may require that the cycle be repeated. Thus, the psychologically healthy individual is one who is able to recognise where constructs have become either too tight or too loose and is able to make a shift in his or her thinking which successfully incorporates new elements.

Personal construct therapy

Like Rogers, Kelly emphasised the importance of the therapist's 'willingness to see the world through the other person's eyes' (Kelly, 1955, p.373). However, the intention in personal construct therapy is to use this to achieve a better understanding of the individual's construct system and to help him or her experiment with new ways of thinking and behaving. Ideally, this process of understanding and reconstruing should help the individual reduce conflicts between core constructs and actual behaviour and should lead to more accurate personal predictions and, therefore, to healthier personal adjustment. A common aim of therapy will be to enable the person to change constructs which are too narrow or too broad in scope.

Initially a person's constructs are explored in order to explain why he or she came for help in the first place. Then, through discussion, an agreement (mutual construction) is formed between therapist and client as to the nature of the problem, its possible cause and likely means of treatment. Constructs may be elicited and explored through discussion or, more formally, through a self-characterisation task or the development of a repertory grid of constructs. A self-characterisation is obtained by asking the person to write about him or herself in the third person as though 'written by a friend' who knows the person 'perhaps better than anyone really could'. Self-characterisations may vary according to which 'self' or role a person sees him or herself in. This exercise helps the therapist explore how the individual perceives him or herself and views his or her place in the world. The repertory grid is a means of representing and analysing individual personal constructs. For example, using repertory grid techniques , Fransella (1972) not only found that stutterers have more elaborate, more easily articulated constructs about what it means 'to be a stutterer' than they have constructs about what it means 'to speak fluently' but also showed that those individuals who linked their personal identity with stuttering were the ones who found it more difficult to reduce their dysfluency. In this research constructs were elicited for the repertory grid by asking the subjects to describe 'the sort of person people see me as being when I am stuttering' and 'the sort of person people see me as when I am NOT stuttering'.

In terms of a 'therapeutic style' the therapist assumes the role of a 'supervisor' who assists the 'research student' with experiments in reconstruing experience and changing behaviour. Different alternatives may be considered, agreed and tried if the first is not effective in solving problems.

One treatment approach which may be used to achieve change is 'fixed role therapy'. In this the therapist may be involved in helping a person evaluate his or her hypotheses/assumptions/constructs by adopting a new role between sessions. To do this, the therapist encourages the individual to make an 'experiment in living' by 'acting' a new role for an agreed period of time. This allows the person to try out a new construct (for example, 'being assertive is better than being passive') and to experience a new self-image (in this case, being assertive) which has not been tried before. As can be seen from this example, the role of the therapist in personal construct therapy is more directive than in client-centred therapy.

In the field of speech pathology, personal construct therapy was originally applied in the treatment of stuttering. As referred to earlier, Fansella (1970, 1972) related personal construct psychology to stuttering by means of the repertory grid test. Her research suggested that stuttering should be seen as a psychological process, not just a behavioural dysfunction, and she has argued that the transition from dysfluency to fluency has to be carried out with care because of its effects on the person, since as the role of fluent speaker develops, then new predictions have to be made and elaborated. During treatment, therefore, therapy works towards creating changes in self-concept (core role constructs), which in turn lead to a reduction in dysfluency (the behaviour).

Since Fansella's pioneering work, personal construct therapy has also been applied in work with children with speech difficulties and their families. In this area, Hayhow (1987) found the approach helpful in relation to several different aspects of clinical work. She writes:

> It clarifies the nature of the relationship between therapist and client; it provides a framework within which to understand the client and the problems

that the client brings to therapy, which in turn leads to assessment and treatment strategies.

(pp.3–4)

Brumfitt and Clarke (1982) have also described the use of personal construct therapy in the rehabilitation of adult brain-injured patients. In these cases an important focus is on the sudden change in core role constructs as a result of trauma. For example, stroke victims suffering from dysphasia have to adjust to this change or loss and also have to cope with having faulty or little communication about their feelings. In such cases the repertory grid may provide a medium through which the therapist assists in the process of self-reconstruction.

For reasons similar to those given concerning stutterers, children and their families, and brain-injured adults, personal construct therapy can also be a relevant approach with other problems, including the treatment and management of dysphonia at those times when the speech pathologist encounters resistance to changing voice, lifestyle or attitude and in work with trans-sexuals and puberphonics.

Evaluation

The brief summary given above of Kelly's personal construct theory and therapy can serve only as an introduction to this treatment approach and is not a comprehensive review. In trying to highlight the most important elements in personal construct therapy, we are aware of a number of important omissions. In itself this illustrates one of the difficulties of becoming a skilled personal construct therapist. Kelly was not only an original thinker and innovator but was extraordinarily rigorous in the development, presentation and elaboration of his theoretical and therapeutic model. His main publication covers two volumes of over a thousand pages and reading the original can be as challenging as reading a text by a major philosopher. Whilst meeting such a challenge may be extremely rewarding in forming a deeper understanding of cognitive psychology and psychotherapy (many leading cognitive therapists, such as Beck, Ellis and others, have acknowledged their debt to Kelly), it should be stressed that it is not an easily accessible nor easily mastered form of treatment. However, as borne out by extensive research, those fully trained in personal construct therapy have at their disposal an extremely versatile means of both understanding and modifying individual cognition and behaviour. The full significance of personal construct therapy can be seen in the fact that, whilst it has developed in a way which has been largely independent of other cognitive–behavioural therapies (Neimeyer, 1986), many of its fundamental principles not only predate these therapeutic models, but continue to form a large part of them.

Behaviour therapy

A major premise of behaviour therapy and social learning theory is that animal and human behaviour is shaped and reinforced by classical and operant conditioning. In the field of speech pathology, this behavioural model has been applied to a range of speech and language disorders including stuttering, voice disorders, articulation and phonological disorders and aphasia (Purser, 1982, Chapter 11).

In treating stutterers, it has been assumed that the stutter is a 'learned response' which was established initially, and continues to be maintained in the present by environmental reinforcement. Therapy aims at disrupting the conditioned response, as well as the reinforcement which maintains it, and to replace this with more appropriate or adaptive behaviour. Therefore, during treatment, fluency is positively reinforced or rewarded – for example, with attention or praise – while dysfluency is not reinforced – for example, if a person produces a dysfluency, they have to stop speaking (or have a 'time-out' from the rewards of speaking) for an agreed period before continuing.

The behavioural model can also be applied to the understanding and treatment of voice disorders. Purser (1982) states that:

> A purely behaviourist approach to dysphonia in the absence of organic damage would be to regard this behaviour as caused and maintained by environmental reinforcement. Functional analysis might reveal the sources of such reinforcement which could then be subject to the usual extinction and shaping procedures.
>
> *(p.306)*

Although only small-scale studies have been made of treating aphasics with operant conditioning (Goodkin, 1969; Ince, 1973, 1976), these appear to have produced beneficial results. In these cases, the treatment has been used as a means of shaping and reinforcing the production of sounds, words and whole sentences. To quote Purser (1982) again:

> Operant programmes attempt to shape behavioural responses in gradual steps by presenting a reduced input and output demand to the individual under reinforcement conditions. Gradually this input and output demand is built up and elaborated under more refined reinforcement conditions. This simplication of input–output structure, together with reinforcement (which may act as feedback information), may be responsible for the progress patients make in this paradigm.
>
> *(p.307)*

Evaluation

The application of simple behaviour therapy principles to the treatment of speech disorders is now an established part of the speech pathologist's therapeutic armoury. However, many speech pathologists feel that this is a rather limited or one-dimensional way of construing and treating speech difficulties. For example, we have already cited the important, if not central, role played by cognitions in maintaining stuttering behaviour (compare Fransella, 1972) and how this should be addressed in treatment. Similarly, our own findings and those of, for example, Aronson (1990a), and House and Andrews (1987, 1988), indicate that while social factors and social reinforcement may be important in the development and maintenance of psychogenic voice disorder, this is only one influence or feature among many others of equal or greater significance. Concerning the application of behaviour therapy to the treatment of aphasia, it should be stressed that while attempts at speech may be positively reinforced, Purser (1982) rightly highlights how a behavioural rationale is limited in this area, since the poor communication is not entirely due to environmental reinforcement.

Because of the difficulties just outlined, many speech pathologists have turned to approaches which incorporate behaviour therapy techniques within a more broadly conceived treatment modality. The wide use of anxiety control training and its application in the treatment of conditions described above is a good example of this trend.

Anxiety control training

Anxiety control training was developed by Snaith (1981), who defined it as follows:

> Essentially it is a technique through which the patient acquires the skill of emotional self-control and is encouraged in the process of cognitive reshaping of destructive or maladaptive attitudes towards himself and his environment.
>
> *(p.213)*

He has stressed, however, that the approach will only be successful when anxiety is the basis of the disorder and when the patient is sufficiently motivated in complying with the practice. The Irritability–Depression–Anxiety (IDA) scale is recommended for use at the initial assessment and at intervals throughout the course of therapy to identify the presence of depression which would affect the success of the programme (Snaith et al., 1978).

The basis of anxiety control training is 'auto-hypnotic or meditative' – often referred to as 'relaxation training', as this is possibly a preferable term for patients. Once the patient is familiar with the relaxation technique, Snaith (1981) suggests introducing imagery which is mildly anxiety provoking while at the same time helping the patient to employ a cognitive–behavioural coping strategy. This procedure is later incorporated into home practice and, over a period of time, greater degrees of anxiety imagery are introduced within the sessions. The emphasis is on regular practice and commitment to the programme while the relaxation skill is developed in the presence of stressful stimuli, both in imagination and in real life. Compliance needs to be encouraged and rewarded with verbal praise by the therapist.

In recent years anxiety control training has become popular with speech pathologists in the UK and there appear to be three main reasons for this. First, it includes autogenic and hypnotic techniques, which are familiar to therapists working with dysfluency and voice disorder. Second, its simplicity and style allow it to be easily incorporated into a therapeutic approach used in speech pathology. Third, it can be adapted to a wide variety of conditions as illustrated below. Turnbull (1987) has described how anxiety control training can be used with stutterers who generally experience anxiety during the act of speaking and for those stutterers where it only occurs in certain speaking situations. She suggests that anxiety control training can help control anxiety in different situations and break the predictive nature of the anxiety triggering an 'automatic stuttering reaction'. She provides examples of 'overt very mild stutterers' who experience considerable anxiety in relation to their stutter and 'more obvious overt stutterers', who would not be described as 'anxious personalities' but who experience increased anxiety in speaking situations.

Anxiety control training has similarly been employed with patients with psychogenic voice disorder as a means of both reducing general anxiety and vocal symptoms and reducing predictive anxiety in specific speaking situations. In these cases it is assumed that the voice disorder itself has created fear and phobia and anxiety control training can be employed to disrupt this pattern of maladaptive predictive behaviour.

Anxiety control training can be used with adults who have acquired neurological conditions as a means of reducing anxiety and negative construing associated with the pressure of speaking. For example, it can help to reduce anxiety about word-retrieval problems or sudden blocks when speaking, or the anxiety provoked by listener reactions to unusual or unclear speech.

Anxiety control training has application for carers, either individually or in support groups, as a means of reducing the anxiety which has arisen as a result of supporting a sick relative, friend or spouse. Coupled with suitable coping strategies, anxiety control training helps carers to cope better with their change in role.

Evaluation

As can be seen, anxiety control training is a versatile treatment technique which has many applications to those conditions found in speech pathology. Its versatility probably arises from its basis in a cognitive–behaviour model of treatment and the exploitation and integration of a number of practical, well proven, treatment strategies. However, despite these positive features, there are a number of limitations associated with anxiety control training which should be highlighted.

While making no claims to be more than a technique for anxiety management, anxiety control training does not compare favourably with procedures like personal construct therapy, which offer wider scope in their approach to understanding the origin and treatment of individual problems. In other words, anxiety control training does not provide a fully comprehensive model for formulating, assessing and treating the many, varied and often complex life problems encountered within the clinic (see, for comparison, the following chapters). This point can be illustrated in two ways. First, while anxiety control training may be extremely valuable as one approach to treating anxiety, there are several other treatment strategies for anxiety associated disorders which the therapist can employ (see Chapter 5 for examples). Second, Snaith has rightly highlighted that anxiety control training has nothing to offer in those cases where symptoms of depression need a focus and he has been careful to screen out this population. In contrast, many of the cognitive–behaviour treatment strategies we will outline in this book were initially developed and successfully used in the treatment of mild-to-moderate depression; see, for example, Beck (1976) and Burns (1980).

Thus, in conclusion, while we can recommend anxiety control training as a specific treatment strategy, it should be stressed that it will not provide the therapist with the conceptual sophistication or breadth which we feel is necessary to respond adaptively and fully to the range and complexity of individual patient needs. In the following chapters we will illustrate how cognitive–behaviour therapy addresses these issues.

Summary

In the course of treating speech disorders the speech pathologist is frequently required to use a range of methods which have their roots in counselling and psychotherapy. In such cases the therapist is concerned with helping and influencing people through psychological techniques. Whilst training colleges do recognise that counselling skills are necessary, the extent to which these are taught varies. In no case does the training course equip the speech pathologist to be a fully competent counsellor. Hence, therapists must look to postgraduate courses to become skilled not only in counselling but also in other psychological therapies. Those who have sought further knowledge and training in this area have been drawn to a wide variety of psychotherapeutic models. However, client-centred counselling, personal construct therapy and behaviour therapy appear to have had the widest influence. Whilst each of these, as well as other therapeutic methods like anxiety control training, has much of value to offer speech pathology, we have also highlighted their particular disadvantages or limitations.

Chapter 3
The Cognitive–Behaviour Model

According to a survey conducted in the USA, cognitive–behaviour therapy has become one of the dominant forces in psychotherapeutic practice (Smith, 1982). Academic publications have shown that this form of treatment can be successfully applied to a wide range of individual problems, including anxiety states (Matthews, 1985), anger and pain management (Novaco, 1975; Meichenbaum and Turk, 1976), mild-to-moderate depression (Rush et al., 1977), alcohol and drug dependence (Gossop, 1985) and obsessive–compulsive disorders (Rachman and Hodgson, 1980; Salkovskis, 1989).

In this chapter we will attempt to give a brief description of what can be considered 'cognitive–behaviour therapy' and show how it is similar to or differs from the psychological approaches described in Chapter 2.

Unlike psychoanalysis – which grew out of Sigmund Freud's work with psychologically disturbed patients in the late nineteenth century – and unlike behaviour therapy – which could be said to have its origin in the early part of the twentieth century with Ivan Pavlov's studies of classical conditioning or J. B. Watson's behavioural psychology – cognitive–behaviour therapy has not developed from the ideas and investigations of a single individual. In fact, there is no clear agreement as to when the principles of cognitive–behaviour therapy were first conceived or used to treat individual problems. A case can even be made for the view that many of its principles were outlined in early Buddhist texts, as well as in other ancient sources such as the writings of the stoic philosopher Epictetus; see, for example, Kwee (1990).

This having been said, it is generally agreed that contemporary cognitive–behavioural systems for treating psychological problems first emerged in the 1950s with George Kelly's personal construct therapy and Albert Ellis's rational–emotive therapy. In the 1960s and 1970s there were several other new developments, with Arnold Lazarus's multimodal therapy, Donald Meichenbaum's cognitive–behaviour modification and Aaron Beck's cognitive therapy the best known and most influential. A book published in the mid-1980s on the cognitive–behavioural approaches to psychotherapy describes ten distinct styles of therapy which fit comfortably within the model (Dryden and Golden, 1986). In addition, since the training of psychologists tends predominantly to emphasise cognitive and behavioural models, many clinical psychologists adopt this model in treatment and draw liberally from different schools of cognitive–behaviour therapy. A study cited by Weishaar and Beck (1986) suggested that in the early 1980s the term 'cognitive–behaviour therapy' described the treatment orientation of about 40% of new psychologists appointed to academic posts in the USA.

Thus, while cognitive–behaviour therapy is not simply a single theoretical model and method of treatment developed by one individual, cognitive–behaviour therapists hold certain assumptions or views in common and tend to adopt similar methods in the treatment of psychological problems. In the following sections we review what we feel to be important or essential features in making an approach 'cognitive–behavioural'.

Phenomenology, self-awareness and self-education

The word 'phenomenology' was coined by the philosopher Edmund Husserl (1895–1938) to describe the philosophical and scientific study of the contents of human consciousness. The term and the general approach continue to have value in contemporary psychology where they are associated with

> ... the view that the phenomena of subjective experience should be studied because behaviour is considered to be determined by how the subject perceives himself and the world ...

> *(Davison and Neale, 1978, p. 648)*

According to Nordby and Hall (1974), a phenomenological analysis is 'the description of the contents of immediate awareness, what is going on in a person's mind right now' (pp.23–24). This emphasis on phenomenology has particular importance for cognitive–behaviour therapy because the therapist assumes that a prime task is understanding the individual's inner world, particularly the way a person makes sense of his or her experiences. In keeping with this view, a large part of the assessment tends to focus on looking at personal beliefs, attributions, concepts, expectations or predictions and the inner or subjective statements which individuals make to themselves about life experiences. Understanding this subjective realm is considered important because of both the emotional and the behavioural changes created by these cognitions.

In the endeavour to assess cognitions an important emphasis is placed on helping the individual increase his or her self-awareness or skill in self-monitoring. Essentially, it is assumed that learning and change occur when the individual observes and then understands the nature of restricting unnecessary or dysfunctional concepts which cause emotional distress. In this way, and unlike many other therapeutic approaches, the therapeutic hour is not considered the sole or main cause of personal change; it is only one hour out of many in which the individual has the opportunity to increase self-awareness and to create personal change. Cognitive–behaviour therapy is, therefore, implicity or explicitly self-educational. To aid this self-educational process, and to gather data, cognitive–behaviour therapists have applied traditional behavioural methodology – observation, diary keeping and target setting – to subjective phenomena as a way of helping individuals observe, record and change cognitive processes.

The holistic orientation

Far from just focusing on cognitions and considering how these affect emotion and behaviour, cognitive–behaviour therapy attempts to be comprehensive or holistic in its orientation. This means understanding as far as possible all the individual factors which may have a bearing on the origin, nature and maintenance of a problem or problems. Being holistic in this way is necessary not only to understand causes but also to find problem solutions.

Cognitive–behaviour therapists have described the most important areas of focus in slightly different ways but there is common agreement on what should be assessed and the major elements which combine to make a whole picture. The approach described by Arnold Lazarus may be a helpful starting point. He uses the term BASIC I.D. as a mnemonic to describe what he believes are the main areas of consideration. BASIC I.D. refers to:

B Behaviour
A Affect or emotion
S Sensation
I Imagery
C Cognition
I. Interpersonal relationships and
D. Drug-related, biological or biophysiological factors.

Kwee and Lazarus (1986) emphasise that the concept of the BASIC I.D. is part of a general systems theory approach to understanding how processes and modalities interact.

> The BASIC I.D. ... is ... a complex of components in dynamic and mutual interaction organised for adaptation. The components are interconnected in a causally connected sequence, and ... not a single modality exists in isolation.
>
> *(pp.325–326)*

Among other things relating to the BASIC I.D. they stress the important concepts of *wholeness, relationship, homoeostasis* and *feedback*. In making these points they illustrate how the cognitive–behavioural approach is concerned, first, with a whole system, second, with the way that different processes interrelate and, third, with the way in which harmony (homoeostasis) should be achieved through circular feedback loops within the system so that even when disruption occurs there is, ideally, an appropriate (i.e. adaptive) readjustment.

Our own attempt at being comprehensive has been to emphasise the importance of understanding the interrelation between cognitions (thoughts and imagery), emotions, physiological reactions, behaviour, the escalation of symptoms through 'negative feedback', interpersonal relationships and life events. The following sections briefly introduce some of the particularities of these individual processes or events and show some ways in which they interact with one another.

Cognitions

From the moment of birth individuals begin absorbing and processing information that will be of value in adapting and surviving in the world. This processing forms the foundation of thinking. With the development of language and more sophisticated abstract patterns of thought, thinking becomes not only a means of explaining the world and making sense of ourselves and our actions, but also a way of solving the often complex problems which we confront in everyday life.

In studying the way we process information, how we know or conceive ideas and how we solve problems, cognitive psychologists have established that much of this is done automatically or unconsciously; see, for example, Williams et al. (1988). Furthermore, they have shown how sometimes preconceptions or the fact that we jump too quickly to conclusions can cause errors in thinking which have a negative emotional impact.

Thinking and feeling

A good example of thought coming to the wrong conclusions and causing emotional distress can be taken from the case of Sidney, a 63-year-old man who had suffered for much of his life from symptoms of anxiety and depression. Having made progress in treatment, he suddenly became quite depressed following the death of a pet cat. Always an individual who strove for perfection, he blamed himself for not taking his cat to the vet and was unable to stop thinking about what he believed was a mistake or failing on his part. When discussing these thoughts, the therapist asked what evidence Sidney could produce to show that (1) he must never make a mistake, that (2) he was uncaring or that (3) he could or should have acted differently.

In the process of exploring his initially unquestioned beliefs, Sidney admitted, first of all, that everyone in the world makes mistakes. Second, he acknowledged that he was certainly not an uncaring person, because he loved his cats and would always take one to the vet if he believed it needed treatment. Third, in thinking it through, it became clearer to him that he did not do so on this occasion because the cat's symptoms did not appear too serious. Finally, he wondered aloud why he was blaming himself alone for not taking the cat to the vet when both his wife and grown-up son were at home and were equally responsible for not acting. The therapist suggested that if other people had not felt it was necessary to take the cat to the vet, this could be further proof that the illness did not appear life-threatening.

By reviewing his thoughts in this way, Sidney was able to conclude with some confidence that he had been jumping to conclusions and distorting or misinterpreting events; there was no evidence for his acting badly and he had no reason to blame himself in the way he had done in recent days. Consequently, his mood lightened. A week later he reported that, while he had continued to experience periods of depression, he had been able to challenge the self-recrimination which produced them, to look at the events 'more clearly' and to think himself out of feeling down.

Sidney also suffered from a number of anxieties concerning his appearance – at times he was very self-conscious about the size of his nose – and he was not comfortable in a number of social situations. Since most people have experienced at least mild anxiety in some social situations, it may be helpful to illustrate the way thoughts influence emotions by using this as the next example.

Social anxiety probably has its origin in concern about self-presentation and fear of being judged harshly by other people. Positive thoughts and images about social situations and the judgement of others may be expected to improve self-confidence and to reduce anxiety, while negative thoughts and images should have the opposite effect. This view has been supported by various research projects, a good example being the conclusions of Bates et al. (1991):

> Consistent with cognitive conceptualisations of social anxiety, the articulated thoughts of anxious males were distinguished by greater focus upon the self in general and by a concentration upon irrational concerns in particu-

lar. In contrast, non-anxious males provided larger proportions of thoughts directed to the environment and in particular, provided more positive thoughts both about other persons and their interactions in general.

(p.91)

In support of a more general connection between negative thinking and emotional disturbance, Bates et al. also cite a review of the research literature which concluded that this was the distinguishing feature of dysfunctional cognition and that an individual's degree of emotional disturbance was reflected in the ratio of negative thinking to positive thinking (Schwartz, 1986). Thus, the general conclusion is that the greater the frequency or intensity of negative thinking in proportion to positive thinking, the greater the emotional disturbance.

The connection between the frequency and intensity of negative thinking and emotional disturbance can be illustrated by the case of Grace, a woman in her late fifties who developed dysphonia a year after the death from cancer of her only son. Ear, nose and throat assessment of her dysphonia showed mild bowing of the vocal cords, characterised by intermittent voice loss, pitch breaks and occasional breathing problems, with no evidence of organic pathology. While substantial gains were achieved through training in vocalisation technique and breath support for speech, her volume of voice remained low and the quality deteriorated further whenever she became emotional. Because of the presence of continued anxiety, her lack of progress with anxiety management techniques and symptoms of depression, she was referred for a psychological assessment. This revealed a wide range of negative thoughts about her abilities or achievements and her lovability or likeability as a person. These thoughts included long-standing negative beliefs about always having been a poor mother to her son because she lacked energy or stamina as a result of her rheumatic heart condition; she believed that a bout of depression when her son was three years old had been too much for her husband to cope with and had caused his problem with alcohol; she believed, thereafter, that she should have done more to help her husband overcome his alcohol abuse; she felt guilty over leaving him shortly before his death about 15 years earlier; she believed that she always made wrong decisions; and she believed that current difficulties in the relationship with her daughter-in-law supported a long-held personal belief that she was someone who was never liked or popular with others. All these beliefs were quite unfounded or irrational. In the course of treatment she came to acknowledge that, despite her physical illness, she had been a competent mother, that her husband really had had 'a weak character' and had put all responsibilities on her, that he had been drinking heavily prior to her period of depression, that she did more than most in staying with him for 16, very difficult, years of marriage, that she had no good reason to feel guilty about leaving him for the sake of her health, that she had made many good decisions during her life, and that her difficulty with her daughter-in-law was an exception rather than a rule in relationships since she had many long-lasting friendships and acquaintances. Challenging and helping her change her many negative beliefs played an important part in reducing her mood disturbance. As her mood became more positive, there was also a noticeable improvement in her quality of voice.

Autonomic and biophysiological changes

What we experience psychologically as emotion is always associated with inherited or innate biological responses, various changes in nervous system activity and other physical changes. This can be readily illustrated with the emotion of anxiety. Feeling anxious is normally accompanied by physical changes such as increases in brain wave activity, adrenalin, oxygen and lactate levels in the blood, sweating, higher blood pressure and heart rate, as well as decreases in galvanic skin resistance, saliva flow and the function of the body's immune system or the ability to fight disease (see, for example, Wallace and Benson, 1972; Van Rood and Goulmy, 1990).

Whilst most cognitive–behaviour therapists recognise that constitutionally the biological system of some individuals may be more sensitive to stress and may thus react more violently under stressful conditions, they also assume that reducing any frightening thoughts which produce the emotional reaction and the associated physical changes would reverse this negative chain of events.

Behavioural changes

Emotional responses are also accompanied by observable behavioural changes. Accompanying the emotion of anxiety for example, we will usually observe most or all of the following: muscular tension; restlessness or agitation; distractibility or difficulty sticking to a task for even short periods of time; hyperventilation or the tendency to breath in a rapid and shallow way using the muscles of the chest or thorax; and phobic avoidance of specific situations.

An appreciation of behavioural changes, how and why these occur and what factors, such as classical and operant conditioning, may maintain these reactions will be important in devising an appropriate programme of treatment. The behavioural aspect of a particular treatment programme will target ways of making positive behavioural changes that will reverse negative responses as well as reactions which have become habitual.

The 'negative spiral'

The changes described in the preceding pages can also lead to other cognitive, emotional, physical and behaviour changes. Increased adrenaline may be experienced subjectively as feeling 'edgy' or 'jumpy'; poor concentration may produce feelings of frustration and irritability which manifest themselves in outbursts of temper; hyperventilation may produce dizziness and tingling in hands and fingers, which can be very disconcerting. These examples show how one process will interact with another in a way which produces a chain of events wherein a negative, ever worsening, trend or 'negative spiral' can be established. For example, a person with a fear of flying becomes anxious initially because of thoughts and images associated with boarding a plane which might crash. These thoughts and images produce various physiological and behavioural changes, e.g. palpitations, rapid breathing and agitation, which stimulate further fears, e.g. fears of not being able to get off, of not being in control, making a fool of oneself or becoming physically ill: 'I'll be locked in. What if these symptoms get worse? What if, once I'm locked in, I can't stand it, go berserk and run amok? I'd feel so embarrassed. My symptoms could get so bad I might not be able to breath. Perhaps my heart will give out.' These thoughts are accompanied by vivid images which also make the anxiety state or the symptoms much worse. Note how one fear (of dying in a plane crash) and the accompanying symptoms have produced other fears which might be categorised as follows:

1. Thoughts and images of being locked in, restricted or trapped.
2. Thoughts and images of the symptoms escalating.
3. Thoughts and images of going mad, berserk or running amok.
4. Thoughts and images of losing control and making a fool of himself.
5. Thoughts and images of dying from either breathing difficulties or from a heart attack.

In the time it took to think the thoughts and have the images the fears have more than quadrupled and created a mental state which has exacerbated the phobic anxiety. From a cognitive–behavioural assessment and treatment perspective, it is important to understand this process and look for the means of reversing a negative trend.

Interpersonal influences and life events

This chapter has tended to focus on the individual and on understanding how individuals make sense of themselves and their worlds, how this information is processed and the effects this can have emotionally, physically and behaviourally. However, each individual exists in a particular historical context and is shaped by various environmental, cultural, political, social, economic and family forces. Although all these may be relevant in understanding any individual, in most cases probably none has greater psychological importance than the influence of family and interpersonal relations.

An example of how important early environmental influences and personal relationships are in shaping personality can be taken from the studies in mothering and infant deprivation. The quite well known experiments conducted by Harry F. Harlow and his team of researchers using infant rhesus monkeys clearly demonstrated how monkeys deprived of normal mothering and socialisation develop severe disturbances which continue into adulthood (Harlow and Zimmerman, 1959). More recent research into mothering and infant deprivation in humans has highlighted the importance to the infant of establishing an early, strong, stable, personal tie or *attachment* to a care giver or care providers. If the care giving is poor or inconsistent or if the bonds of attachment are broken or suddenly disrupted, the child will very likely experience *separation anxiety*. If there is separation from the main care giver and the child is also placed in a strange environment, the anxiety and disturbance will be intensified. Studies of individuals who experienced maternal deprivation and long-lasting, multiple separation experiences – particularly if these occur in infancy – suggest that these experiences produce long-term consequences including vulnerability to anxiety and depression, relationship difficulties, delinquency and adult conduct disorders (Rutter, 1975).

These studies illustrate the important influence early environmental and personal relationships can have on individuals, affecting the way they think about their worlds, and how well they adapt to various personal, emotional and social demands. Thus, from a cognitive–behavioural perspective, it is important to consider developmental and family influences or early life events which may be contributing to the individual's current condition.

The influence of recent life events

While events in childhood may predispose the individual to psychological or emotional difficulties, when assessing an adult the therapist also needs to take account of recent life events. This is particularly important because research not only suggests that negative early life experiences increase the individual's vulnerability to emotional disorder but also indicates that emotional disturbance is commonly associated with (or brought out by) stressful life events in the individual's recent past. For example, studies have shown that women who, before eleven years of age, have lost their mothers through death are prone to develop severe depression when confronting unfavourable life events in adulthood (Brown and Harris, 1978).

Life events, such as the death of a spouse, divorce, marital separation, a prison sentence, death of a close family member, retirement, sexual difficulties and so on, rank highly in terms of the stress they create, while other events, such as changes in social activities, changes in the number of family gatherings, taking a vacation or celebrating Christmas are not, generally, considered highly stressful (Holmes and Rahe, 1967). However, research like that of Brown and Harris described above suggests that it is not just the *severity* but also the *number* of life events which is important. Thus, even less stressful or minor life events are associated with psychological and physical illness when enough of them occur in reasonable close succession within a period of 12 months.

We can also note that many life events that are generally considered positive turn out to be negative or to contain negative elements. A simple example is a vacation which proved to be disappointing and, for one reason or another, rather exhausting. Another example is that, whereas most would consider marriage a positive life event, it usually involves a number of negative and stressful elements such as major changes in personal habits as well as increased personal and financial responsibilities. Thus, evaluating the *number* and *intensity* of recent life events or events surrounding the onset of a particularly disorder is extremely important. From the cognitive–behavioural viewpoint, crucial considerations will be whether individuals recognise the presence of stress, the way they interpret it and how they respond emotionally and behaviourally. For example, a newly wed man, having gone into marriage without considering the debit side of the contract, may abruptly become aware of changes in routine, restrictions on his social life, increased responsibilities and extended financial commitment. He may conclude that his wife wants to restrict his freedom or does not understand his needs or, simply, that to marry was a mistake; he may feel trapped and resentful about being asked to contribute his share to the marriage; he may appear moody and withdrawn and begin a pattern of staying out late, drinking with old friends. Here we can see how an individual response to a life event (the marriage), which contains a mixture of positive and negative qualities, can establish a destructive behavioural trend which affects not only the person concerned but also those to whom he is most closely related.

Common assessment and treatment procedures

In the following chapters we will look in detail at cognitive–behavioural approaches to assessment and treatment but it may be helpful to introduce briefly some features relating to these activities which have not been highlighted so far. In doing so, we hope to provide a more complete picture of what is involved in adopting a cognitive–behavioural orientation when working with clients.

A sound therapeutic relationship

As in other forms of counselling and psychotherapy, cognitive–behaviour therapists recognise that an important requirement of treatment is creating the right atmosphere in the session so that the client feels able to trust the therapist and to be open and honest about intimate feelings or embarrassing secrets. Client confidentiality is obviously important in establishing this trust, but the therapist also needs skill in demonstrating appropriate levels of concern, sympathy and non-judgemental respect for the client. The client-centred therapeutic triad of *unconditional warmth* or *regard, empathy* and *genuineness* is extremely important (Rogers, 1961).

Collaboration and self-help

Providing the right therapeutic relationship should also include conveying the philosophy that sessions are essentially about self-help being achieved through therapist/client collaboration. Here the emphasis is on respecting the client's resources, including the ability to learn new skills and to change old patterns of thought and behaviour. The person is encouraged to see the sessions as opportunities to deepen self-understanding, to acquire tactics and skills for personal development and to focus on what he or she can do to create change right now and in the days to follow. One distinct advantage of this philosophy and of making the treatment model explicit is that, in the eyes of the client, the therapist is divested of mystery and power and the focus of control and the focus of change are placed in the hands of the client. In principle, this should also reduce the well-known tendency of clients to become either dependent on their therapist or addicted to weekly treatment.

Assessing the ABCs

Although methods of assessment have much in common with other forms of data collection, such as medical and psychiatric history taking, as a generally rule they tend to focus more particularly or in greater detail on an analysis and interpretation of what have been called *the ABCs of dysfunctional thoughts and behaviours*. The ABCs stand for the antecedent or activating event (A), the following belief or behaviour (B), and the consequence (C) either emotionally or in terms of negative or positive reinforcement. Essentially, the therapist is asking: 'What *life events* trigger these particular thoughts or actions?' and 'What is the person *thinking* and *doing* which creates and maintains undesirable emotional and behavioural reactions?' These considerations are necessary if the *origin* and *maintenance* of any problem are to be understood and changed.

Making the treatment model explicit

Unlike most other psychotherapies, the cognitive–behavioural approach attempts to make the nature and rationale of treatment as clear as possible. Different therapists approach this in different ways but it usually involves an explanation about the interrelation between thoughts, emotions and behaviour, interpretations aimed at helping the person make sense of symptoms (for example, giving a description of autonomic arousal and the fight-or-flight response to a person suffering from attacks of panic) and explaining the rationale behind specific therapeutic procedures.

An emphasis on self-instruction

Having earlier described the nature of thinking and the way it attempts to give meaning to experiences and to provide solutions to problems, we also need to add that thinking has another role in helping us conduct our lives. This is the role it plays in directing our actions toward particular goals. Commands or instructions to ourselves may be of importance in the following ways: First of all, self-commands are frequently helpful in talking ourselves through a difficult situation (e.g. 'Whether or not my boss thinks I deserve a pay rise, I believe I've earned it and I'm going to ask for it. Anyway, I've nothing to lose by asking.'). Second, giving self-commands helps inhibit undesirable or impulsive behaviour (e.g. 'He's not listening to my case. Don't lose your cool. Don't thump the table. That won't help. He'll just think I'm a jerk.').

Because of the way thoughts influence emotions and motivation and help inhibit impulsive behaviour, a universal procedure in cognitive–behaviour therapy is helping individuals become more skilled in saying the right things to themselves. This is done in various ways but often includes the therapist highlighting or challenging unhelpful or negative thoughts, giving guidance in ways to think more positively or rationally, using role playing or behavioural rehearsal as a means of initial practice and setting agreed targets in order to develop the skill of positive self-instruction.

A structured problem–solution focus

Sessions tend to be more structured than is the case in traditional counselling and psychotherapy. The therapist directs attention to the present or to recent events in order to assess problems and develop potential solutions, which are then acted on or tried out through specific target setting. Target setting typically takes two forms: first, homework exercises designed to gather more information (for example, keeping a daily record sheet of situations which trigger negative thoughts) and, second, asking the client to experiment with or try out alternative thoughts and/or behaviours. Once treatment is embarked on, a typical session usually involves three areas of focus:

1. Evaluation of homework from the previous week.
2. Time for exploring anything new or pressing which the client wants to discuss and to consider the need for additional treatment strategies.
3. Preparation of homework or targets for the coming week.

Ideally, the structure should provide a framework or orientation for the therapist, but in order for it not to interfere with the therapeutic relationship and atmosphere, the formula should not be one which is rigidly adhered to.

A time-limited treatment contract

Whereas most traditional psychotherapies are unstructured or open ended in not setting limits on the number of treatment sessions, cognitive–behaviour therapists frequently offer a time-limited treatment contract or a specified number of contacts. A course of treatment of between eight and a maximum of 20 sessions would be fairly representative. A common practice is to start by offering six or eight sessions, at the conclusion of which progress is reviewed and any further sessions offered as appropriate. The time between later sessions is often extended gradually so that, eventually, meetings take the form of a follow-up. Thus the client receives an intense course of treatment over about two months and then gradually learns to cope with less frequent support. Knowing that treatment is time limited can increase patient motivation and this, as well as gradually extending the time between later sessions, can be a factor which reduces patient dependence. However, as in other therapies, it is important that therapists prepare their clients for ending treatment, reminding them of how many sessions remain and exploring their feelings about concluding the agreed contract. Obviously, some clients express fears about coping without their newly found source of help, but reducing frequency of, and eventually ending, sessions can be presented by the therapist as a means of further confidence building and practice in independent self-help. Furthermore, the client should be informed that another assessment and treatment contract can be arranged if a crisis or problem occurs at any time in the future.

Summary

In summary we can say that the cognitive–behavioural model is phenomenological in highlighting the value of self-monitoring in data collection and holistic in emphasizing the presence of important causal connections between psychosocial, biological and behavioural events or processes. The main areas of focus in assessment are on understanding the relationship between environmental life events, personal relationships, thoughts and images and emotional, physiological and behavioural reactions. Particular stress is, however, put on the way that emotional disturbance and associated difficulties are created or exacerbated by errors in thinking and problem solving.

Therapy emphasises establishing a sound therapeutic relationship, demystification, collaboration, self-help, active data collection, altering irrational or negative beliefs, self-instruction, cognitive and behavioural target setting and multiple treatment strategies. Therapeutic methods are made as explicit as possible and treatment contracts tend to be brief in duration.

Chapter 4
Cognitive–Behavioural Assessment Procedures

Conveying to another person the principles of cognitive–behavioural interviewing can be difficult if that person is not familiar with the psychological model and the way assessment will need to be adapted for individual differences and for different types of psychological disorder. Even those who from training and experience in their profession are extremely skilled in history taking often fail to ask the right questions or gather the necessary information to formulate working hypotheses. They may not know how to ask clients to record both thoughts and behaviours and they may not be sure what, in terms of intervention, follows from the data collected. Hence, anyone wishing to conduct an adequate cognitive–behavioural assessment first of all needs a good basic understanding of the psychological model and, second, needs to know how to gather the right sort of information, which will lead to the most appropriate treatment plan. Hopefully, Chapter 3 has provided an introduction to the cognitive–behavioural model and has given some indication of how this orientation 'prescribes' what questions need asking and what data need collecting in order for a programme of treatment to be formulated. Thus, it should be possible to move straight on to describing the general assessment orientation, some diagnostic issues, the use of assessment forms, methods of eliciting automatic thoughts and methods of implementing daily record sheets as part of the overall means of gathering and collating information.

Listening, observing and formulating hypotheses

In Chapter 3 we stressed how important it is to establish a good rapport with clients. Much of this comes from the therapist's skill in listening. Clients will not feel that there is empathy, acceptance, understanding and support unless they have a sense that what they are trying to convey is being heard and appreciated. Since many thoughts and feelings which clients bring to therapy are only half formulated and understood, are difficult to express or articulate and are often being described for the first time, the therapist will need to listen for clues in what clients are trying to describe and also to have a sensitive ear and keen eye for underlying themes or hidden messages.

For example, if a woman suffering from anxiety symptoms describes in an apparently matter-of-fact way how she achieved her childhood ambition to be a dancer, gave this up after having a child, then had some success as a model until work dried up and that she now works in a mundane job, the interviewer may speculate about the emotional effect of losses of meaning, purpose, fulfilment and a positive identity associated with the changes described. Although the description of these events may have appeared matter-of-fact, the emotion surrounding them may have been conveyed, non-verbally, through momentary changes in vocalisation such as a slight tremble in voice or hesitation over words, tension around the face, moistening of the eyes, changes in posture or increased tension, agitation of, or fidgeting with, the fingers, hands, arms, legs or feet. Thus the skilful interviewer must be able to listen, observe and formulate hypotheses for testing. Very few people are naturally able to do more than one thing at a time and for these three skills to operate successfully in parallel usually requires a good deal of practice and experience. Thus the state of mind of the interviewer must be alert and attentive as well as curious, puzzled, questioning, intuitive and open to inspiration, while also speculating about and synthesising information. The great difficulty for most people is to do all this at the same time. It is all too easy to forget to listen for possible hidden meaning, to miss a gesture or to get caught in speculation and formulation and, as a consequence, not hear or see something essential to understanding. However, knowing the importance and combined value of these skills, and remembering to prioritise them whenever embarking on an assessment, will lead – with practice over time – to better interviewing and data collection.

Questioning

In addition to having the attributes described in the last section, the skilled interviewer needs to know the best way to elicit the information he or she needs from the client. This can only be achieved by being skilled in the art of questioning, not only being aware of *what* questions should be asked but *how* the questions should be put to the client. Most readers of this book will probably be speech and language therapists or other health professionals with an interest in psychogenic voice disorder; from their training they will be aware of what have been termed *closed questions* (those questions to which the answer will be either 'yes' or 'no', e.g. 'did you feel anxious when thinking about discussing your feelings with your husband?') and *open questions* (the answers to which required a freer description or elaboration in the person's own words and terms, e.g. 'What sort of feelings did you experience when you thought about confronting your husband?'). Both types of question have value: the open questions to limit any bias in thinking and questioning on the part of the interviewer and for maximum information, and the closed questions for collecting specific or precise detail, which may be important. In the following example, an interviewer uses three open questions followed by two closed questions to obtain the most data:

Interviewer:	What were you feeling when you thought about confronting your husband?
Client:	Anxious.
Interviewer:	What was that like?
Client:	Churning in my stomach. Sweating. Tense. Dry mouth.
Interviewer:	Anything else?
Client:	Not that I recall.
Interviewer:	Was your heart racing?
Client:	Yes, it certainly was.
Interviewer:	Did you notice whether you were breathing differently?
Client:	No. Wait a minute. It became very rapid – like I needed more air or something.

Describing the importance of employing a combination of open and closed questioning, Wilson et al. (1989) noted the following:

> There may be occasions when you realise that a more open question was required after asking a closed question. In such situations, it is often helpful to ask the question again with some slight modification. It is especially important to ascertain whether the person has actually answered the question that you intended, or whether the client has answered 'another question' due either to a misunderstanding of the question as stated or to some other factors such as avoidance of certain issues.
>
> *(p. 10)*

As Wilson et al. also stress, it is particularly important to give care to the choice of words, to avoid jargon,

> to judge the level of vocabulary that is appropriate for an individual client, and to tailor your language accordingly.
>
> *(p. 10)*

The value of reflection

One skill which can be valuable in collecting more information, as well as in formulating hypotheses, is for the interviewer to voice his or her thoughts out loud in response to something which has just been said by the client. Here the interviewer rephrases what has just been mentioned in order to encourage further elaboration on the subject and to help the interviewee consider further what he or she has just said. For example: 'So, from what you were saying, there seemed to be various changes going on at home in the months before your voice started to play up?'; 'When you were saying that, it looked to me as though you felt quite angry about what happened?' Statements such as these are an implicit formulation of the therapist's thinking, indicating that a connection is being made between life changes or emotions and voice loss. Many people with psychogenic voice loss will previously not have made connections of this sort. In considering such questions they may begin to explore the link between life stresses, anger and voice deterioration. Thus, reflection of this sort demonstrates that the interviewer is listening empathically as well as making specific connections. It may stimulate further discussion of important details surrounding voice loss and also begin the important process of information giving or patient education. In summing up and presenting a formulation to the client at the end of the interview, the therapist reflects back in a more comprehensive and formal way, but we will describe this practice later in this chapter.

Focusing the interview

As we shall see, while a history of developmental and personal experiences will be invaluable, a distinguishing feature of cognitive–behavioural interviewing is that it tends to focus the main attention on more recent circumstances and current difficulties. Thus, the majority of questions will be aimed at eliciting a detailed and accurate description of recent relationships, problems, minor and major life events and cognitive, emotional, behavioural and physical reactions to these experiences. An advantage in directing attention to more recent events is that people's recall is often more accurate and detailed. Also, once a detailed analysis of recent events has been made, it is often easier to make comparisons with the more remote but formative experiences of childhood. For example, detailed questioning about a recent event may reveal that the voice loss was associated with a circumstance where there was conflict over expressing an unpopular view or an opinion. If a therapist has not considered it previously, he or she may then wonder what the family attitudes were to the expression of views and ask questions around this area. If the topic of expressing views in childhood has been touched on previously, the client and therapist may make a connection between the recent event and certain experiences of parenting, such as having a rigid father who would not tolerate being questioned or criticised. In this way, the focus and the questioning deepen understanding of the psychological process behind a specific problem.

Another reason for focusing on more recent events is that it should not be assumed that childhood experiences always play the most important part in the creation of a difficulty. In the above example, it could be that the client has had parents who tolerated the expression of views and who reacted positively to criticism. However, the client may now be in a relationship with a person who would react violently or punitively to criticism. The client wants and knows how to express an unpopular view, but is in conflict because of fears of precipitating a negative reaction from the partner and fears of causing a deterioration in a relationship which in other ways is valued and rewarding.

The above example highlights the need on the part of the interviewer not to be prejudiced by his or her theories about the cause of the client's difficulty; in this case, not to assume that all psychological problems are formed in childhood. Preconceptions and theories are valuable only as hypotheses and the enormous value of good questioning is that it is usually the best means available of testing whether there are data to support a particular interpretation or whether the evidence suggests that the theory should be abandoned in preference for a more likely formulation.

Important information

Basic information

Most readers will be familiar with the procedure of recording basic information. Typically, this includes a record number, date of interview, name of client, client's date of birth, address, telephone number, occupation, marital status, the source of the referral and the name and address of the general practitioner.

General information and assessment of the current problem

Although the order in which the information is gathered may vary and different therapists approach data collection in slightly different ways, questions will focus around the following areas.

The reason(s) for referral

The main complaint(s) and symptom(s), frequency and severity
Since patients with psychogenic voice disorder may tend to concentrate on their voice loss, it will be important to probe for other symptoms that are commonly stress related such as difficulty in sleeping, increased frequency of headaches/migraine, physical tension, attacks of panic, hyperventilation, etc.

A history of presenting complaint (including any treatment)

Family background

- Relationship with mother and father, type of person, their age, health, occupation, current contact, etc.

- Number of siblings, ages and order of birth, type of relationship(s), current contact, etc.
- General home environment.
- Other significant figures (e.g. grandparents, aunts, foster parents).
- Life events (e.g. separation/divorce of parents, death of sibling, etc.).

Personal history

- Early development, family and social relationships.
- Personality as a child (e.g. shy/outgoing; confident/nervous, etc.).
- Personality prior to symptom onset.
- Health (including psychiatric as well as medical illness and treatment).
- Education. Attitude to school. Qualifications and whether or not academic potential was fulfilled.
- Employment history.
- Personal and sexual relationships.
- Marriage(s) and children.
- Current social circumstances.
- Alcohol and drug use.
- Police record.

The above list highlights areas which should be covered in order to be certain that information that may be important in understanding the disorder is not omitted. However, while details of family background and personal history can be invaluable, there will be many occasions when it is not possible or necessary to cover everything. One example is when a client sets the agenda. This commonly happens when the client is particularly distressed about a certain issue in his or her life and the interviewer feels it would be inappropriate and insensitive to begin asking questions about topics which may seem irrelevant to what the client wishes to talk about. The good interviewer will allow him or herself to be led by the patient, but will keep the above list in mind and ask questions from it when the opportunity arises.

The most common difficulty in a busy voice clinic will be not having enough time to be as comprehensive as we have suggested. However, whilst not ideal, in these situations it is possible to elicit some, if not all, of the most important material with a few well focused questions. Aronson (1990b) has highlighted an interviewing approach that we would wholly endorse for its speed and efficiency. He states:

> The following questions have worked well in getting patients to talk about themselves. 'Think back to when your voice trouble started. What was going on at that time that might have upset you? Is there anyone at home or at work whom you have been having problems with, such as your partner, children, parents, in-laws, colleagues, or supervisors? Have you had trouble

expressing your feelings to these people? Have you been concerned about your health or the health of your family, or career, or your finances?'

(p.289)

In gathering the basic information, personal details and history, it is essential to integrate this information with the therapeutic framework or model. In Chapter 3 we described this model as 'holistic' and we will return to this theme in order to describe its relevance in the art of assessment.

The overarching holistic framework

In order to conduct a good cognitive–behavioural interview, it is extremely important to have the ability to construe the information within a holistic framework and to appreciate how different interpersonal and intrapersonal processes influence one another. We suggest that as a general guide the diagram in Figure 4.1 is comprehensive enough for the purpose of considering causality and formulating strategies for intervention. To illustrate the importance in interviewing of considering the interrelation between the five processes shown in the figure, we will give three examples.

John, a student in his early twenties meets an acquaintance who invites him to a party the following Saturday. His immediate thought is 'I won't know any people. I'm useless at starting conversations. I am going to stumble over words and make a fool of myself, etc.' and he pictures people looking at him and laughing. These thoughts and images of making a fool of himself have an emotional impact and,

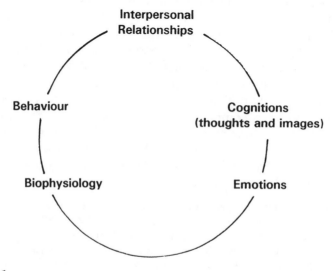

Figure 4.1

because of the anxiety and physical tension which are then evoked, he does not go to the party. Here we can see how the meeting with an acquaintance was an event that triggered specific thoughts, feelings and uncomfortable physical changes (autonomic arousal, muscular tension) and why, because of these reactions, he avoids the party. Note that if, upon receiving the invitation, his thoughts had been 'Great, I can meet new people. I'll have a good time and enjoy myself', his emotional, physical and behavioural reactions would have all been positive rather than negative.

In our second case, Martha, a woman in her fifties, presented with a protracted anxiety state. Assessment showed that in the year prior to seeking help there had been a number of life changes and bereavements which had very probably contributed to her condition. However, her more acute state of anxiety could be traced to a recent event. She was standing behind the counter in the confectionery kiosk where she worked and was about to serve a customer. Suddenly, the woman lurched towards her with outstretched hands. Martha recoiled in shock and, a moment later, realised that the customer was having an epileptic fit.

An assessment of Martha's cognitions surrounding the event was very fruitful in making sense of her anxiety state. Her first thoughts were that she was being attacked and about to be strangled. This produced a flood of fear. She then realised that the woman was not about to strangle her but was having an epileptic fit. Most people would feel some sense of relief at this realisation because they would no longer feel threatened, but this was not the case for Martha. She had had a life-long fear of illness and all things to do with illness and this event, coming as it did when she was struggling to cope with the bereavements of the past year, left her very shaken. In the following days her state of anxiety remained very high: she was extremely tense physically, was restless and agitated, found it difficult to concentrate, frequently hyperventilated, felt dizzy, developed nervous diarrhoea and was unable to go in to work. When she was asked about her thoughts concerning these changes in herself, she reported that in general she feared she was going mad and that, because of the diarrhoea, she was quite convinced that she had bowel cancer. Understandably, these interpretations greatly increased her anxiety state and made it difficult for her to regain any mental, emotional and physical equilibrium. The process of change can be depicted diagrammatically (Figure 4.2) in a form which follows a downward and negative spiral of anxiety.

Our third case is Sarah, a community nurse in her thirties, who developed dysphonia and who was assessed to be mildly depressed as well as to be suffering from a number of home- and work-related stresses. One particular source of interpersonal stress concerned her relationship with her husband, who was domineering and authoritarian.

Figure 4.2

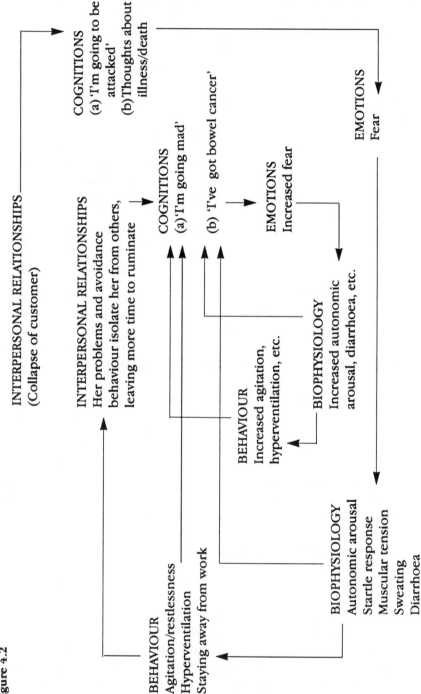

He not only left her with all the responsibility for family decisions, but gave her no indication that he appreciated the hard work she put into running both her job and their home. Although she wanted to express her dissatisfaction about these matters, she was unable to do so, largely because he made her feel powerless and inadequate. She also feared expressing her views because she believed that her husband would not listen, that she did not have the persuasive powers to make him change and that any comments would only anger him and make matters worse. Furthermore, she held the view that 'a good wife tries to please her husband and make him happy'. This strongly held belief created a dilemma: criticising her husband would certainly displease him and make him unhappy and it therefore followed that if she did this she would not be 'a good wife'. Not unexpectedly, her situation and psychological conflict had an emotional impact, causing feelings of anxiety, helplessness and mild depression. Physically, her emotional state manifested itself in muscular tension, dysphonia and disturbed sleep. Her attempts to please her husband and her physical agitation, or restlessness, were manifested behaviourally in obsessional tidiness and cleanliness around the home.

In Sarah's case the difficult relationship with her partner, the dilemma created by the thought that 'a good wife always pleases her husband' and the conflict over speaking out were important factors in her feeling anxious and depressed, developing musculoskeletal tension and dysphonia, as well as becoming obsessional about housework. Never allowing herself to rest would aggravate and probably exacerbate many of her symptoms. The less she rested the more she would become physically exhausted and tense. This additional stress and increase in musculoskeletal tension would inhibit possible progress with voice therapy or cause her voice to deteriorate further. We can also speculate that if she were then to attribute the reason for lack of progress to a serious physical condition (e.g. throat cancer), she would, like Martha in the previous example, have an additional cause of stress to affect her cognitions (worries about dying), emotions (heightened fear), physical state (autonomic arousal) and behaviour (visits to specialist for a second opinion, etc.).

The ABCs

In Chapter 3 we have already described the importance in assessment of considering what have been called the ABCs – the Antecedent or Activating event, the Belief and Behavioural Consequences for the person. The ABCs are probably most clearly illustrated in the second example where the Antecedent event (the customer's epileptic fit) caused physiological and Behavioural changes (e.g. hyperventilation, agitation, diarrhoea, increased frequency of visiting the toilet) and changes in *Beliefs* ('I'm going mad', 'I have bowel cancer'), the *Consequence* of which was an increased, protracted anxiety state. An understanding of how these individual processes are activated and how they influence or stimulate other, related, processes will aid the therapist in developing a comprehensive or multifaceted treatment programme. In this example the therapeutic strategies which would result from the assessment would include helping the patient change the thought 'I've got bowel cancer' to thoughts such as 'I've got diarrhoea because I've got a nervous stomach. This was caused by the fright I had with that customer. I have had diarrhoea before when I've been nervous about exams, so being nervous is a believable explanation for this symptom'. In addition, therapy would target relaxation training to reduce autonomic arousal and physical tension, breath retraining to control hyperventilation and a graded desensitisation programme with training in rapid relaxation to help Martha start back at work.

The three Ps

Some therapists find that a helpful alternative to conceptualising problems in ABC terms is to consider them in the form of *Predisposing*, *Precipitating* and *Perpetuating* factors. If the third example above, of acute anxiety, is used as an example, a formulation of this kind might look as follows.

Predisposing factors

Long-standing difficult in assertiveness and expressing views. Holding the view that 'a good wife always pleases her husband'.

Precipitating factors

Marriage to a man who is domineering. Increased feelings of powerlessness. Not expressing feelings over a recent domestic issue and holding in frustration, anger and resentment.

Perpetuating factors

All the above, plus belief that husband will not listen to her views and that speaking out will make things worse. Autonomic arousal, agitation and increased effort to please through doing more at home.

As can be seen in this particular example, there may be overlap between the predisposing, precipitating and perpetuating factors However the 'three Ps' provide a helpful framework for thinking about both the causes of the problem and the requirement of treatment.

Eliminating disorders unlikely to respond to cognitive–behaviour therapy

The initial interview and information about personal history should provide the therapist with enough material to decide whether the patient is likely to benefit from cognitive–behaviour therapy. For reasons we will outline, there are certainly two psychological conditions associated with psychogenic voice disorder which are highly resistant to any form of psychological therapy: hysterical conversion syndrome and severe personality disorder.

Hysterical conversion disorder

Where there is a non-organic, complete loss of voice accompanied by a marked lack of concern or *la belle indifférence*, as well as a denial of having any life stresses and an apparent lack of effort to use the voice, e.g. being content to mouth the words, treatment will be difficult on two fronts. First, the indifference displayed about the loss of voice will make it difficult to motivate the patient and it is highly unlikely that he or she will comply with various treatment strategies. In fact, if it is assumed that in these cases the voice disorder provides an unconscious means of avoiding anxiety and that the displayed indifference is also a defence against feeling anxious, making any changes would mean that the patient would have to recognise or acknowledge the cause of his or her anxiety, discard avoidance strategies or abandon his or her 'solution' and face all the discomfort that this entails. In this way the primary rewards of losing the voice, coupled with any secondary gain – such as increased attention and support from others – would have to be sacrificed. Probably for these reasons, it has been found extremely difficult to break through the very strong sense of denial which is manifest in these cases. Second, conducting cognitive–behaviour therapy requires that the therapist and patient engage in a dialogue involving an analysis of the patient's thoughts and feelings and, while the aphonic remains defensive and complacent, therapy is impossible. Fortunately, as reported by House and Andrews (1987), clearly diagnosed hysterical conversion disorder occurs in only 4–5% of people with psychogenic voice disorder.

Personality disorder

According to the third edition of the American *Diagnostic and Statistical Manual of Mental Disorders* (DSM-III, American Psychiatric Association, 1980, p.305), the diagnostic term 'personality disorder' can be applied to individuals whose traits are inflexible and maladaptive and cause either significant impairment in social and occupational functioning or subjective distress.

(cited by Davison and Neale, 1982, p.272)

DSM-III describes ten varieties of personality disorder, but there are real difficulties in making a reliable diagnosis – even for experts – as well as disagreement on both the validity of using these categories and making the assumption that the condition is associated with specific personality traits. Thus we will not attempt a comprehensive description of diagnostic guidelines. What we will highlight are features which are commonly associated with personality disorder and which can make success in therapy unlikely. The first of these is poor reality testing; the person may be a dreamer, who is easily lost in an extremely vivid fantasy life, or someone who has an uncertain image of him or herself or who has a confused identity. Another feature of poor reality testing may be that the person does not consider the consequences of actions in a way that would usually be judged as normal. In this he or she can be said to be lacking a conscience; such people often manifest antisocial behaviour and will frequently have been in trouble with the law or will be found living on the fringes of society. These individuals tend to be unreliable and have difficulty with relationships and they may be mildly paranoid or aloof, or use others for their own ends. They may be highly unpredictable in moods and attitudes and behave impulsively without due regard to their own welfare or that of others. Often this behaviour is related to high levels of pleasure seeking and to being oriented to gaining excitement. However, whilst some individuals will be impulsive and pleasure seeking, others may be quite the opposite, demonstrating either overly perfectionistic behaviour and rigidity or a stubborn or highly oppositional nature, the passivity of which masks an angry or aggressive individual. These characteristics create obvious difficulties in personal relationships and many people with these characteristics will be constantly seeking attention and may show manipulative or seductive tendencies. Superficially they may appear to be attractive or charming individuals, but beneath this they are easily revealed as non-genuine, self-centred, and exploitive. The craving for attention or adoration may show itself in exaggerated or fantastical views of their own importance. Finally, a poorly developed positive self-image or self-concept may, in some cases, manifest itself as an extreme lack of confidence or as overdependence on others, which can be extremely demanding for all concerned with their welfare. As might be expected with such high levels of emotional instability, it is not uncommon to find that these patients have a history of (sometimes multiple) suicide attempts.

What we hope to have highlighted here is that, whilst some of these characteristics may be present in a milder form in many patients who are eminently treatable with both speech and cognitive–behaviour therapy, the greater the number of the above 'symptoms' and the greater the evidence that these features are both pervasive and long-standing, the less confidence we would have about being able to help the individual make appropriate or positive change.

Questionnaires

In addition to the data collection described earlier, the therapist wishing to gather more data concerning the client's background and condition can use a specifically designed assessment form. For example, speech pathologists may be familiar with using Snaith's (1981) Irritability–Anxiety–Depression scale as a screening devise. Alternatively, where the interviewer wishes to assess the degree of depression, the Beck Depression Inventory (Beck and Steer, 1987) may be used. This is a brief questionnaire (taking about 5–10 minutes to complete) with 21 items measuring negative attitudes, somatic disturbance and performance impairment, as well as providing an overall depression score. Beck and Steer (1990) have also developed a brief questionnaire to measure anxiety. However, it should be borne in mind that symptoms of anxiety and depression commonly co-exist and also that, because the questionnaires have been developed for use with psychiatric populations, scores should be interpreted cautiously when other groups of patients are assessed.

If the interviewer wishes to assess levels of social confidence and assertiveness, he or she could use an inventory such as the 30-item assertiveness schedule developed by Rathus (1973). However, although this gives a summed total score of assertiveness, like most measures of social competence it provides very little specific information about how a person will respond in different social situations. While it may be helpful to know that a person is generally low on assertiveness or that, despite the presence of social anxiety, he or she does not always avoid certain social situations, this knowledge is fairly limited. Since individuals react in various ways in different social situations (the same person may be confident and relaxed in one setting but anxious and verbally inhibited in another), it will be more valuable to have details about these situationally specific responses in order to plan treatment. Thus, although cognitive–behaviour therapists may use questionnaires, the above example shows why they tend to treat each case as unique and to emphasise the use of a carefully detailed assessment of individual differences and reactions in specific situations.

Since wrong thinking can be an important cause of anxiety and depression, it may be valuable to understand the nature and type of dysfunctional thoughts which are at the heart of the problem. Although these can be elicited through careful interviewing, a very helpful questionnaire is the Dysfunctional Attitude Scale (DAS). A self-scoring version with guidelines on how to interpret the results has been published by Burns (1980). Essentially, this scale measures the individual's psychological strengths and areas of emotional vulnerability along seven dimensions entitled Approval, Love, Achievement, Perfectionism, Entitlement, Omnipotence and Autonomy. For example, a person who overvalues the importance or necessity of always obtaining approval, love, success and perfection would have a negative score on the first four scales. He or she would be considered emotionally vulnerable in these areas since it is unrealistic to expect that approval, love, success and perfection are either one's by right or wishing or that they can be attained on every occasion or in all situations.

The value of using a scale like the Dysfunctional Attitude Scale can be illustrated by referring again to the case of Sarah, the community nurse who suffered from dysphonia. Her Dysfunctional Attitude Scale profile showed very high negative scores suggesting emotional vulnerability in the area of approval, love and omnipotence. She not only expected or needed a great deal of approval and love from others, but she also had a very distorted view of her personal influence on the people and events surrounding her; essentially she tended to hold herself responsible for either events or the reactions of others that were largely or completely outside the realm of her personal influence or control. For example, responding to the Dysfunctional Attitude Scale, she strongly agreed that: 'I should assume responsibility for how people feel and behave if they are close to me'; 'To be a good, worthwhile, moral person, I must try to help everyone who needs it'; 'I should be able to please everybody'.

This dysfunctional attitude has been called 'omnipotence' because, as shown above, the person tends to exaggerate the extent of their personal influence. Another way of referring to this tendency in thinking has been to describe it as 'a personalisation error'. In this case, Sarah had a strong tendency to blame herself for the actions and attitudes of others when these were not really within her control or realm of influence. Because of this particular tendency in her thinking, Sarah spent a great deal of time being self-critical, condemning herself for various things which did not go right and suffering a great deal of unnecessary guilt, all of which lowered her mood or made her feel depressed.

In this case and most others, however, this information is still rather limited as it simply describes a general tendency in thinking. It does not provide a full picture of the *specific* challenges encountered by the person in daily life, nor give us details of the personal reactions to these events. This information will be invaluable in understanding an individual case and in developing the appropriate, individually tailored, treatment programme. However, it is difficult to obtain this information simply through interviewing and questionnaires. What is required is a method of current or ongoing data collection. The usual way of gathering more detailed information is to ask the clients to collect the data themselves on a prescribed record sheet.

Daily record sheets and ongoing assessment

Completing a daily record sheet is rather like keeping a diary. However, it is a diary with an imposed structure so that the required information is recorded in an organised or consistent way. For example, during the first step in data collection, a daily record sheet may be set out as shown in Figure 4.3. When enough data have been collected for the problem reaction to be clearly understood and to suggest a particular treatment strategy, the daily record sheet can be modified to include a specific therapy target. However, it should not be assumed at this stage that the assessment phase is over. When treatment is begun important new material may be collected and often this leads to modifications in the treatment approach. This change from assessment into what we can call the treatment and ongoing assessment phase can be illustrated with the following example.

Date	Situation	Reaction
		(what you thought and what you did)

Figure 4.3

In the case described earlier, Sarah was asked to keep a three-column record under the following headings. The *Situation*, *The Worry* and *The Positive Response* (thought and/or action). As illustrated by the sample in Figure 4.4, her records over the following weeks showed that she commonly developed a positive behavioural response or solution as a way of reducing worries. However, detailed questioning showed that, in the main, she had great difficulty accepting that her action was good enough. Because of her tendency to think in an 'omnipotent' way, she not only believed that she should have done more but was unable to stop worrying about what could have been done if circumstances were different. Thus, while her 'positive solution' went some way in reducing her initial worry and would have been sufficient for most people, it did not significantly alter the time she spent emersed in self-critical and negative thoughts. By focusing on this tendency, it was then possible for the therapist to point out to the patient the important way in which a belief of this sort would affect mood and cause depressive or anxious feelings. Understanding how a particular belief affects mood can then lead to the development of an appropriate cognitive–behavioural treatment programme. In this case the patient was guided in how to change a negative, unproductive or unhelpful belief by using the following statement to herself whenever she had taken a positive action but the 'omniscient' worries still intruded: 'I've done my best; no-one else would do more; it's done; I'll let it go', and then to follow this by occupying herself with whatever was appropriate at that time in a further attempt to disrupt the tendency to dwell on what was worrying her. The example illustrates how good assessment is both ongoing and can lead to improved treatment.

The Situation	The Worry	The Positive Response
Mr C's home visit from the optician.	That Mr C won't hear the door knocker because of the builder's noise and the noise from his O_2 supply.	Phoned optician to alert him to the situation.

Figure 4.4

The daily record form can be modified in a number of ways in order either to collect particular information or to treat different conditions. For example, a patient suffering from an obsessional condition in which upsetting images frequently intrude into consciousness could be asked to begin recording the situations in which images occur. The aim here is to look for things that have triggered an image. If an appreciation of the cause of the images is reached, the patient can then be helped to record not only situations and negative images or thoughts but, in the course of increasing awareness and deepening understanding, to begin using positive thoughts and actions as a means of becoming less distressed by the images and/or to gain more control over them. Figure 4.5 shows a sample from a daily record sheet of a patient who has an obsessional fear of harming her child and who is some weeks into treatment. Hopefully this example will show how, in the midst of treatment, the record keeping has stimulated a better understanding of the processes involved in the problem.

Patients often need some guidance or help with their data collection and in implementing the treatment strategy and it can be helpful if the initial form includes some examples of what the person is expected to record. For example, see Figure 4.6.

In the case of individuals suffering from dysphonia, it will be particularly important to collect a record of the time of day the condition

Day/Time	Situation	Negative image/thought	Positive image/thought
Friday 8.30 am	In work. Customer came in with his baby. Cute little girl. Looked same age as Tom [her baby]	What if I burn his baby with a cigarette?	First I became aware of cigarette because we were all smoking and the smoke was blowing all over the baby. First thought was the poor little thing can't breath, then I just thought of burning the baby because of the habit of thinking CIGARETTE [i.e. cigarette = danger], then the bad thought of burning the baby with it. I didn't panic so much [because of this review and explanation to myself].
Sat 10.00 am	At home	Walking in bathroom and [had image of] finding baby floating in bath [and] thinking [that] I had put him there.	Started to panic about the thought of baby floating face down in bath. Realised the thought triggered off because I became aware of bathwater running and not wanting the bath water to overflow - relaxed myself and realised I was just panicking over image of baby floating in bath, then told myself there is no way I could put him in the bath without knowing. Just frightening myself again with the bad thought that I might not be able to tell the difference [between an image and reality] when I know I can. Just worried about his safety, so I am judging myself, e.g. am I in some way a danger to him when I know I am not. Just love him and trying to protect him from everything ...
Sat 11.25	Getting ready to go to work	Panicky because I am late, also because [boyfriend] John will be on his own with the baby. Started to get bad thoughts [about harming the baby] as well.	Told myself to relax. It's not the end of the world if am late. John will be OK with the baby and as for the bad thoughts they are just a habit I have to break. I know I only get them because I worry about his safety all the time. I just love him and never want anything to happen to him and it won't, it's just me being silly.
Sun 9.00 am	At home. Drinking cup of tea	Fleeting thought of spilling tea on baby.	Could see this one coming. Another habit. Just relax and let it go.
Mon 6.45	At home. Feeding baby	Thoughts of throwing tea over baby.	First looked at myself. I never realised how much I panic feeding baby before. Just relaxed and [told myself] not [to] let the bad thought bother me. When baby cries I start to panic. Probably I think I have got to stop him crying just in case it winds me up and I lose my temper. I just relax and it doesn't bother me.

Figure 4.5

Date	Situation	Negative autonomic thoughts	Positive alternatives
	Car won't start and I am late for work	My boss will be angry. It won't look good arriving late. He'll think I'm lazy.	I shouldn't assume it will look bad to arrive late or that my boss will be angry or think I'm lazy. I have a very good record for time keeping and I have a valid excuse.

Figure 4.6

either worsens or improves. An alternative to collecting the information under headings like those above can be to provide patients with a prepared sheet showing the days and hours in the week (Figure 4.7). In its simplest form the patient is instructed to place a tick or a cross in each box to show whether during that hour the voice was mainly good or bad and to make a mental note of what was happening at these times. Instead of using a tick or a cross, data collection can be enhanced by providing a five-point scoring key so that the patient can score the severity of the problem.

The disadvantage of this approach is that it does not provide very reliable details about the situations and thoughts associated with positive or negative changes in the voice disorder. Events and associated thoughts become more vague with the passing of time and many people

RECORD SHEET RECORDING VOICE QUALITY

To be kept hourly for seven days. Please mark as accurately as you can on this scale:

0 = no voice
1 = almost no voice
2 = poor
3 = almost normal
4 = normal voice

Leave blank if you do not use your voice.

	Monday	Tuesday	Wednesday	Thursday	Friday	Saturday	Sunday
6-7							
7-8							
8-9							
9-10							
10-11							
11-12							
12-1							
1-2							
2-3							
3-4							
4-5							
5-6							
6-7							
7-8							
8-9							
9-10							
10-11							
11-12							

Note voice from the time you wake up to the time you go to bed.

Figure 4.7

need a lot of guidance on how to be aware of what they are thinking. However, these difficulties are reduced to some extent if the patient has a good memory, is good at introspection and is being seen at least once a week, and if the therapist is skilled in questioning in a way which elicits the information required. Despite its drawbacks, the approach also has some advantages over other forms of record keeping. First, it provides a simple and reasonably accurate means of assessing the frequency and severity of the voice disorder. Second, when used over time from pre- to post-intervention, it should provide a measure of treatment outcome. Third, this method may increase the patient's ability to monitor his or her voice, as well as the circumstances in which it is either good or bad. Fourth, it can provide concrete evidence either of progress or of why there is no progress. The pattern of frequency and severity may be seen by looking at the record and, if necessary, the scores can be placed on a graph, thus providing both patient and therapist with a much clearer picture of just how much progress is being made. In cases where progress has been slow, discovering that the graph shows a gradual decline in the frequency and severity of symptoms can boost the patient's flagging morale.

Ending the initial interview

The way in which the initial interview is ended is an important consideration. The interviewer should remember to ask the patient whether he or she feels there is anything important which has not been covered so far. The end of a session can be a good time to ask this question, because, at this point, the patient is likely to be feeling at least a little more at ease. If, throughout the interview, the interviewer has appeared to be genuinely concerned, empathic and accepting, the patient may now feel ready to go into issues which would have been difficult to discuss at the outset.

There will be those occasions where it is clear that the patient has found the interview emotionally demanding. He or she may have never confided in anyone before or may have suffered an important bereavement in recent months. Perhaps the patient has described events which he or she would rather forget or has been tearful and may regret showing emotion in front of a stranger. In situations of this sort, the therapist should find a way of showing that he or she recognises how demanding the interview has been. The therapist may choose to thank the client for sharing his or her thoughts or being so open and for being prepared to go through something which has proved so uncomfortable.

Alternatively, the therapist may apologise for having to ask questions which were clearly upsetting and at the conclusion, may say 'I'm sorry I've had to ask you so many questions. I can understand how, at times, it's been a quite difficult hour'. A simple comment like this can help the client feel the ordeal was worth while. This will be particularly so if the therapist then adds that it has been helpful in formulating some ideas about the cause of the problem and how it can be treated.

Even if the interview has not appeared to be emotionally demanding for the patient, most people find that attending hospital and consulting a specialist is stressful in itself. They will be looking for answers to their difficulties and hoping for reassurance. Thus, the interviewer should make every effort to meet these needs. One of the best ways to achieve this is for the interviewer to give a brief summary of what has been covered in the session, selecting what appear to be the important explanatory or causal factors in the condition and suggesting that while future meetings will probably add more detail to the picture, it is possible at this stage to offer a tentative interpretation or formulation. If, throughout the interview, the therapist has been conscious of thinking in terms of the overarching holistic model and has been asking questions around life events, interpersonal relationships, cognitions, emotions, physical symptoms and behavioural reactions, he or she will usually find that it is not too difficult to make the right connections and to offer a formulation based on the gathered information. The formulation should be given in simple terms and with as many illustrations as possible to help the patient comprehend what is being conveyed. For example, when talking about the relationship between muscular tension and voice loss, the therapist might manually squeeze his or her own throat to show how this pressure distorts the voice, or when describing how a tendency to hyperventilate causes dizziness, the therapist might ask the patient whether he or she has ever felt light headed after deep breathing, for example blowing up balloons.

In presenting a psychological interpretation, it is important to reassure the patient that the therapist is not suggesting that the problem is 'all in the mind' or that the patient is of unsound mind or mentally unbalanced. Misunderstanding of this sort can easily arise, particularly when the speech pathologist implies that a referral to a psychologist may be necessary. Again, this issue is best dealt with when the formulation is summarised and by presenting clear examples. One way to do this would be to highlight the fact that, while people usually cope well with a reasonable amount or short periods of stress, they are often adversely affected emotionally and physically when stresses become multiple, protracted or intense. Just as physical conditions like a headache or an upset stomach can be caused by worry and stress, so can loss of voice, since the voice is particularly sensitive to emotion. The assessor can then add that a psychological assessment and psychological view of voice loss is concerned with understanding in some depth the life stresses, worries and emotions causing the voice loss and with finding practical strategies to reduce these stresses.

Finally, the interviewer should provide the patient with some idea of what will be offered, including the fact that treatment will be time-limited. Many cognitive–behaviour therapists use this moment to give the patient a brief summary of the treatment model and to describe what this implies for therapy. Since, in the majority of cases of psychogenic voice disorder, there will be stressful interpersonal relationships, the therapist will probably emphasise the role of autonomic arousal in situations of conflict, will mention the value of using anxiety management techniques and of training in assertiveness or the expression of views and will then move on to describing the value of collecting current data and how this can be done by keeping a daily record of such things as stressful events, thoughts, emotions, behavioural reactions and voice quality. In presenting this information the therapist also conveys something of the collaborative nature of treatment.

Obviously, each case is different and ending the assessment session will vary accordingly. However, the interviewer will find that the following general rules should be a helpful guide to how the assessment interview should be concluded:

1. Thanking the patient.
2. Asking whether there is anything important the patient wishes to add.
3. Presenting a tentative formulation.
4. Giving information about the treatment approach or what this entails.

On those occasions where the assessment suggests that the problem is unlikely to respond to cognitive–behavioural treatment, the therapist is faced with the unenviable task of informing the patient that nothing can be offered. At these times the rule of thanking the patient will still apply, but the challenge will be to break the bad news in a way that shows empathy and understanding for the patient's dashed hopes of receiving help. The interviewer has to find a way of being empathic and supportive while breaking the news gently but clearly. Most people find that breaking bad news is difficult. Therefore, to reduce any problems that this entails, the therapist can ask a colleague to help him or her role-play giving bad news as well as the different patient reactions that can be anticipated. Such practice and feedback should increase the skills the therapist already has in carrying out this difficult task and, if role reversal is used, this will also give insight into how it feels to be the patient.

Although being far from comprehensive, the above should provide the reader with a general introduction to cognitive–behavioural assessment procedures. We hope to have covered the most important points and the more commonly used approaches. However, since there can be many variations within the above structure, the reader may find it helpful at some stage to consult the chapters on assessment procedures in Stern and Drummond (1991) and Wilson et al. (1989), both of which describe procedures that can be employed in the assessment and treatment of a variety of psychological conditions.

Summary

Conducting an appropriate cognitive–behavioural assessment is only possible when the therapist has established a good rapport with the client and when he or she has developed the important skills of listening and observing as well as formulating tentative hypotheses. This requires having a state of mind which we have described as alert, attentive and intuitive, while at the same time speculating about and synthesising information. The interviewer will need to be skilled in the art of questioning and should be alert to the way theories and preconceptions will colour interpretations. Good questioning should be used to gather further information to either support or reject a formulation.

It is important to know about the client's personal history and experiences and to focus attention on current circumstances, recent life events, difficulties and stresses. A priority will be assessing the relationship between interpersonal, cognitive, emotional, biophysiological and behavioural processes and evaluating how these relate to problem maintenance and treatment considerations. The interviewer should also be cognisant of those voice-disorder patients who are unlikely to benefit from cognitive–behaviour therapy and should gain enough information in order to make a decision as to whether or not a course of treatment will be useful. A standardised assessment procedure involving questionnaires may be employed in order to gain more specific or detailed information. In addition, cognitive–behavioural assessment employs extensive use of daily record sheets to gather information which is not easily or reliably obtained in the interview or through questionnaires.

As a general rule the therapist should end the initial interview by finding a way of thanking the patient for his or her cooperation, should then present a tentative formulation and, in those cases where treatment is being offered, should conclude with a description of the therapy model and an outline of what treatment entails.

Chapter 5
Cognitive–Behavioural
Treatment Approaches

Since cognitive–behaviour therapy has been adapted and applied in the treatment of a great many, vastly different psychological problems, it would be impossible in one chapter to cover meaningfully the many techniques which have evolved within this form of therapy. Fortunately for the reader seeking an introduction to how cognitive–behaviour therapy can be applied in the context of treating psychogenic voice disorder, it should be possible to confine our discussion to certain areas and still provide a reasonably comprehensive review of what strategies will be valuable in the majority of cases. Table 5.1 lists the strategies the therapist will often find helpful in treating patients with voice loss.

As we have shown in Chapter 1, a number of features appear to be commonly associated with psychogenic voice disorder. First, the most frequently noted and most easily observable feature in this condition is that the patient suffers from a state of anxiety or demonstrates a number of anxiety symptoms such as muscular tension, rigid posture, physical agitation, dry throat, difficulties in swallowing – because it feels as though the throat is tight or has a lump in it – and sweaty palms. Second, but in relation to the first, the psychogenic voice disorder usually follows either an event of acute stress or stress over a long period. Third, the stress and anxiety have frequently been related to the following: problematic interpersonal relationships and marital difficulties (including sexual difficulties); overcommitment in terms of carrying the main burden of responsibility in the family or in failing to set appropriate personal limits; inhibition from expressing views and anger, or experiencing a conflict over speaking out, and feelings of relative helplessness and powerlessness surrounding the ability to change the (patient's) situation. By focusing on these areas, which are usually associated with psychogenic voice disorder, we should be able to illustrate those cognitive–behavioural treatment strategies which will be most commonly employed and which have been found to be useful in therapy.

Table 5.1 Cognitive–behavioural strategies of value in treating patients with voice loss

---

Uncovering negative cognitions

Highlighting unproductive patterns of behaviour

Exploring cognitive–behavioural problem-solving strategies

Implementing specific techniques designed to create cognitive–behavioural change
    e.g. recording thoughts, prior, during and after an event; questioning the unproductive nature of certain types of worry; confronting tendencies to use 'musts' or 'shoulds' or negative predictions; training in positive self-instruction, restricting worry to a half-hour period

Anxiety and stress management training
    e.g. training in the skills of monitoring tension and applying cognitive–behavioural methods of rapid stress control

Target setting

Record keeping

Role playing

Training in interpersonal communication skills

Considering ways to increase the rewards within a relationship

Assertion training
    e.g. considering and practising expressing views, setting limits, standing up for rights, requesting fair treatment, etc.

Feedback and positive reinforcement

Structured programmes using the principles of systematic desensitisation and operant conditioning

---

Anxiety state

A state of anxiety can be easily identified by reports of subjective change and observable physical and behavioural features. People will usually report *emotional disturbances*, variously labelled 'anxiety', 'fearfulness' and 'panic', and these feelings may be accompanied by: more *visceral sensations* of inner restlessness, nervous stomach and lose bowels; *physical changes* such as a dry mouth, sweaty palms, raised heart rate, musculoskeletal tension and an increased rate of breathing; *mental and behavioural changes* such as poor concentration or being easily distracted, intrusive negative thoughts, irritability or outburst of anger, and difficulty sleeping. Most people will recognise having experienced some, if not all, of these symptoms at some time in their lives. In most cases such experiences will be uncomfortable but not so intense or protracted as to feel intolerable or overwhelming in their effect on the normal ability to cope.

Anxiety can be seen as the in-built 'alarm' which 'rings' when we feel physically, personally or psychologically threatened. We intuit danger and the intrusion of anxiety into consciousness makes us fully alert or awake and prepared for defence. At an instinctive or primitive level the mind and body are responding rapidly to danger and preparing to ward off an attack or to run quickly away. The reflex has therefore been termed 'the fight-or-flight response'. Since in some dangerous situations it is better to become motionlessness (e.g. when near a dangerous wild animal which has not seen you or precariously near the edge of a steep drop), this is more accurately called 'the freeze–fight–flight response'. The reaction of 'freezing' also explains why some people become 'rooted to the spot' when frightened.

Understanding the instinctive or reflexive nature of an anxiety reaction and the flight-or-flight response helps us to make sense of why anxiety is accompanied by the symptoms described earlier. When one is threatened and preparing mentally and physically for danger there is a sudden release of adrenaline into the blood stream. Additional adrenaline in the blood increases heart rate and produces feelings of restlessness, etc. Adrenaline needs to be combined with oxygen in order to create energy within the body cells and muscles and additional oxygen is acquired by increasing the breathing rate. Hence, the tendency to overbreath or hyperventilate. In preparing to freeze, fight or flee the adrenaline and oxygenated blood flow into major muscles, which become tensed in preparation for defence. This explains the feature of musculoskeletal tension found in anxiety conditions. Other physical symptoms can be explained as part of the survival reaction. For example, bowels become loose because if an animal defaecates it will be lighter and able to run faster. Similarly, if the animal or human is sweaty the body is not only cooled during strenuous exercise, but may be slippery and more difficult to hold if grasped.

In most situations of physical danger people respond and the adrenaline and oxygen are burned up in the process. Although people are left feeling somewhat shaken, the mental and physical changes quickly reverse. However, when a person is in a situation of intense or protracted stress (i.e. physical/personal threat), the biological changes continue to be activated without a resolution. The consequence of this is that the person is left in a state of physical and psychological distress.

Anxiety management training

Anxiety and stress management training is a core skill in cognitive–behavioural treatment and is practised in one form or another by all exponents of this branch of therapy. Although there are variations and differences in emphasis, most therapists stress the importance of training the patient in physical relaxation techniques. One exception is rational–emotive therapy, which rarely uses physical relaxation training and places more emphasis on teaching clients that they can learn to tolerate the unpleasant affects of stress (Dryden and Ellis, 1988). While recognising the validity of Ellis's argument that training in relaxation may distract the client from discovering that the essential cause of anxiety springs from cognitive distortions, we take a more traditional cognitive–behavioural approach to anxiety management. This can be described as systematically eclectic or multimodal in its treatment orientation and is an approach which draws liberally on any valid strategy which may reduce symptoms and increase an individual's sense of personal control. While there may be a number of ways to achieve this, we have chosen to describe one particular approach. This approach was chosen for a number of reasons. First, it was developed over a number of years by the first author from extensive experience in treating a wide range of patients with anxiety symptoms; second, it has frequently been used in our treatment of dysphonic patients; third, it draws liberally on a variety of cognitive–behavioural strategies and should be a good introduction to the general principles of anxiety management training; finally, as the method is relatively straightforward and simple enough to be used in the form of a self-help audio-tape and booklet treatment programme (Butcher, 1989), it should be reasonably easy for non-psychologists to learn and apply. Those wishing to consider alternative approaches which we would recommend should consult Meichenbaum (1977) or Jaremko (1986) for a description of stress inoculation training, Mitchell (1987) for simple relaxation training and Snaith (1981) for anxiety control training.

Progressive muscular relaxation

Physical relaxation is usually the foundation of stress management training. Many relaxation techniques currently in use are adaptations or shortened versions of a method developed by Jacobson (1938). In Jacobson's procedure the individual is systematically taught to tense and relax the body's major musculoskeletal muscles. Speech and language therapists will be familiar with these principles through their own training and the applications of relaxation methods in the treatment of various speech disorders. The abbreviated version of progressive muscular relaxation employed by the first author in stress management training takes about 12 minutes to complete. Brevity has some advantages over longer methods of relaxation in that it is easier for most people to find this amount of time in which to practice in a day, there is less to learn, and it also reduces the chances of 'practice fatigue' or boredom which can lower motivation. The majority of patients report being able to achieve a noticeable difference in their level of relaxation when first instructed and almost all report further progress with repeated practice. Prior to teaching progressive muscular relaxation it is important to provide the patient with information about autonomic arousal and the fight-or-flight response, as well as a rationale for teaching progressive muscular relaxation. This information must be couched in a simple language. For example, the rationale for learning progressive muscular relaxation can be summed up as follows: A normal baby is born with the capacity to relax and breath diaphragmatically. If this ability has been lost or covered over by bad habits or muscular tension and thoracic (chest) breathing, it is simply a matter of rediscovering an old or innate skill. Rediscovering how to relax can be achieved through learning progressive muscular relaxation. Progressive muscular relaxation practice should increase our skills in being aware of tension and in distinguishing between muscular tension and relaxation. Regular practice not only gives relief from physical tension, but should lead to increased skill in recognising subtle or early signs of tension.

There are some individuals who are unable to relax or who have a negative reaction and respond by feeling more anxious. While this is not common, it is best to warn that this occasionally happens and to provide a possible explanation. One explanation could be that such people have been so tense for so long that the sensation of relaxation is difficult to rediscover or has become so unfamiliar or alien that it feels frightening. Another explanation is that – as in the case of patients where there are buried or suppressed emotions – tension and a 'busy mind' have kept feelings at bay and relaxation allows unwelcome emotions to surface.

To carry out progressive muscular relaxation clients should sit or lie in a comfortable position in a room where they will not be interrupted. In order to reduce distraction further and to aid their focus on subjective and physical changes, they are instructed to close their eyes before beginning the exercises. With the exception of the tension and relaxation of the neck and legs, all exercises are repeated once. If there is any physical reason why an exercise will cause pain, clients are instructed to omit this exercise or do it gently. With each exercise the tension or relaxation is held for a few moments before moving on to the next stage. People are frequently instructed to 'be aware of the sensation of tension (or relaxation) and to notice the contrast between tension and relaxation'. The 12 steps in the procedure are as follows:

1. Clenching the hands into tight fists, holding this for a moment while being aware of this sensation, and then releasing the tension. Repeat.
2. Clenching hands into fists, bringing fists up to the shoulders so that arms are bent and tense throughout, holding for a moment, then releasing the tension by slowly dropping the arms and uncurling the fingers. Repeat.
3. Wrinkling the forehead into a worried frown, holding a moment before allowing the brow to relax and become 'smooth and soft'. Repeat.
4. Screwing up the eyes by pressing down with the eyelids. Releasing the tension. Repeat.
5. Tensing the lower half of the face by pressing the lips together tightly. Releasing the tension. Repeat.
6. Turning the head slowly as far as to the right as possible, holding a moment, then turning it slowly around as far to the left as possible, holding a moment, bringing the head back to the centre, then slowly lowering it forward so that the chin presses into the chest and the muscles can be felt stretching along the back of the neck, holding a moment before returning the head to a normal, relaxed, upright position.
7. Lifting the shoulders as high as possible, being sure not to tense the arms in order to assist this but to keep them limp and relaxed. (When the shoulders have relaxed, the client is asked to see if they can drop their shoulders even further.) Repeat.
8. Arching or bowing the back by gently pushing forward with the stomach and back with the shoulders, then releasing the tension. Repeat.
9. Taking a slow, deep diaphragmatic breath by pushing out the stomach, rather than the chest, and, after holding a moment, releasing the breath as slowly as possible. Repeat.
10. Tensing or knotting the stomach, then releasing the tension. Repeat.
11. Tensing the legs by (a) pushing downward with the heels, holding a moment and relaxing, (b) pushing down with the toes, holding a moment and relaxing, (c) stretching the toes and feet upward or back towards the shins, holding and relaxing.
12. When these exercises have been completed, the client is asked to go back over each group of muscles in order to see if they are still relaxed or whether any tension has returned. The instructions are as follows:

Feel the relaxation in your hands and fingers; your wrists; the forearm and upper arm. See if you can relax even further – if there is any tension just let go of it ... Feel the relaxation in your forehead; round the eyes and eyelids; your cheeks and lips and jaw. If you feel any tension, just let go of it ... Feel the relaxation around your neck and deep down in your shoulders and shoulderblades. See if you can drop your shoulders even further ... Feel the relaxation in your lower back; in the slow rhythm of your breathing; in your stomach; and then feel the relaxation spreading down from your body into your legs; your thighs; calves; ankles; feet; and right to the tips of your toes ... You should now be completely relaxed ... Notice how pleasant relaxation feels and how it contrasts with the sensation of tension ... Just enjoy the relaxation for a few moments ... Now, slowly rouse yourself up to go about your everyday activities. Try not to lose this sense of deep muscular relaxation. Watch out for tension returning. If you notice an increase in muscular tension, just practice letting go of it and see if you can recapture the sensation of deep relaxation.

Rapid stress control

It is one thing to be informed about the nature of anxiety and to be able to relax under ideal conditions, but quite another to achieve relaxation quickly or maintain it under stressful circumstances. Cognitive–behaviour therapists have developed ways of systematically teaching how this can be done. In the self-help course referred to earlier (Butcher, 1989), the programme contains a booklet which gives information on understanding anxiety and tension, learning diaphragmatic breathing, how to relax with progressive muscular relaxation, and how to stay relaxed through a combination of rapid stress-control techniques. Side 1 of the prerecorded cassette, which accompanies the booklet, takes the listener through the progressive muscular relaxation and Side 2 gives repeated practice in the four steps involved in rapid stress control: *self-observation, positive self-instruction, slow diaphragmatic breathing* and *rapid relaxation.*

Self-observation

Self-observation requires that people become aware of the physical and mental stress associated with tension and anxiety. They need to increase the frequency with which they check for signs of muscular tension and whether this tension is associated in any way with negative thinking. If anxiety can be caught before it escalates, it is usually easier to control. To increase the frequency of self-observation and to speed up the creation of a good habit, a simple behavioural strategy is employed: the client is provided with a small red dot to stick on the face of his or her watch; whenever this is noticed, it acts as a reminder to the client to observe his or her physical and mental state. Clients are also encouraged to adapt this ploy to other activities or situations. For example, they might place the red dot (or another reminder such as a small card with '?' on it) around the home or work environment, putting it on a mirror or desk or anywhere likely to catch the eye and stimulate self-observation. (To avoid the tendency not to notice the dot or card after a while, the client is encouraged to move it to other places from time to time.) Another variation can be to use the red stop signal on traffic lights as a stimulus to self-monitoring when driving in traffic.

Positive self-instruction

The use of self-instruction was introduced and briefly described in Chapter 3. However, to explain fully the reasons for using positive self-instruction as a therapeutic strategy, it will be necessary to go into some detail about negative systems of belief and negative self-statements.

Research by cognitive psychologists has indicated that in our every-day use of thought we frequently employ what have been called *schemas*. These are extremely stable and enduring patterns of thinking which develop in childhood and through which we continue to view the world as adults. Schemas are often unconscious or outside awareness, but when an event triggers or activates a schema, our thoughts and emotions become dominated by its influence. For example, a student whose thinking is shaped by a general schema that he is intellectually inferior will automatically interpret a forthcoming assessment as 'too difficult to learn' and predict that he can never pass the examination. Understandably, this schema will produce a good deal of emotional anxiety. Schemas can influence our thinking in a wide variety of ways and in different situations or circumstances. Some idea of this can be conveyed by referring to the Schema Questionnaire developed by Young and Brown (1990) which has 14 types of dysfunctional beliefs subsumed under the general categories of *disconnection* (e.g. beliefs associated with mistrust, social relation), *undesirability* (e.g. beliefs about unlovability), *autonomy* (e.g. beliefs concerning inability to be independent); *restricted self-expression* (e.g. beliefs about the necessity of not expressing emotions); and *impaired limits* (e.g. unreasonable beliefs about the need to be unrestricted by others or beliefs about having insufficient self-control).

If, in self-monitoring, people notice that there are specific negative thoughts and/or images which are causing anxiety, they are encouraged to question both the *validity* and the *necessity* of such thoughts and images and to seek positive alternatives. In the above example of the student making himself anxious with negative interpretations about his ability to learn his chosen subject and negative predictions about passing his test, the aim would be to help him become more critical of these assumptions and to develop more rational interpretations (e.g. 'The subject may be difficult but it is not impossible to learn') and predictions (e.g. 'Why jump to the conclusion that I will fail? I've learned difficult subjects in the past and I've always passed when I've done enough preparation. I should, therefore, predict that I can do it again.')

In Aaron Beck's cognitive therapy clients are encouraged to be as objective as they can about their thoughts and to do this in a systematic way, asking the following sorts of questions:

1. *What is the evidence?*
   What evidence do I have to support my thoughts?
   What evidence do I have against them?
2. *What alternative views are there?*
   How would someone else view this situation?
   How would I have viewed it before I had problems?
   What evidence do I have to back these alternatives?
3. *What is the effect of thinking the way I do?*
   Does it help me?
   What would be the effect of looking at things less negatively?
4. *What thinking error am I making?*
   Am I thinking in all-or-nothing terms?
   Am I condemning myself as a total person on the basis of a single event?
   Am I concentrating on my weaknesses and forgetting my strengths?
   Am I blaming myself for something that is not my fault?
   Am I taking something personally which has little or nothing to do with me?
   Am I expecting myself to be perfect?
   Am I using a double standard – how would I view someone else in my situation?
   Am I paying attention only to the black side of things?
   Am I over-estimating the chances of a disaster?
   Am I exaggerating the importance of events?
   Am I fretting about the way things ought to be instead of accepting and dealing with them as they come?
   Am I predicting the future instead of experimenting with it?
5. *What action can I take?*
   What can I do to change my situation?
   Am I overlooking solutions to problems on the assumption that they won't work?
   What can I do test out the validity of my rational answers?

The founder of rational–emotive therapy, Albert Ellis, has noted that the common cause of anxiety lies in two tendencies in thinking: first, thoughts associated with exaggerating any personal performance or situation in terms of its required level of attainment or its level of importance and, second, thoughts which minimise one's ability to tolerate discomfort (Dryden and Ellis, 1988). Usually, both categories of anxiety-producing thoughts contain generalisations and self-exaltations typically involving 'shoulds', 'musts', 'oughts' and 'nevers' – 'I should never be rejected by anyone'; 'I must be successful to be a worthy person'; 'I ought never to be upset' and 'I will never be able to stand this discomfort'. Note that this last is another 'must' since it reflects the view 'that comfort and comfortable life conditions must exist' (Dryden and Ellis, 1988, p.221).

One thing which all forms of cognitive–behaviour therapy have in common is that clients are encouraged to act much as a scientist would or should in observing the validity of their thoughts. Thoughts are seen as hypotheses which should be challenged or tested and abandoned if found wanting. If, on observation, the thought 'I should never be rejected by anyone' is recognised as unrealistic or untenable because it is impossible for anyone to go through life being loved and accepted by everyone, the person could then begin using positive self-instruction of the following sort: 'Well, I don't like/love everyone I meet, so why should I expect everyone to like me? People have different preferences in what they look for in a person they want as a friend or a lover, so if I'm rejected I should assume that's all that's happened. I shouldn't exaggerate the importance of what's happened and assume that there is something terrible wrong or unlikeable about me to have caused it. Also, I am not going to overgeneralise and conclude that because one person has rejected me then everyone will do so.'

With the thought 'I must be successful to be a worthy person', people should be expected to define what they mean by 'success', to question whether they have accepted a cultural stereotype (for example, the typical Western concept of success is unknown in some cultures, where a person can attach most success to themselves by being good at gardening and cultivating vegetables), to consider alternative ways of measuring success, to question in a similar way what is meant by a 'worthy person' and to consider either how the person can be 'successful' and not 'worthy' (e.g. Richard Nixon, Idi Amin, Sadham Hussain, Robert Maxwell) or to consider people who are not successful in worldly terms but may be considered worthy people.

At the end of this assessment people should be able to develop a number of statements they can make to themselves about 'success' and 'worthiness' that will be more positive than the original self-statement. In all cases, if helpful, these new positive thoughts can be written on a small card which can be carried in a pocket or handbag and taken out when necessary to act as a reminder of the method of replacing irrational thoughts with rational thinking.

The psychologist Donald Meichenbaum has not only highlighted and researched the way that self-statements influence emotion and behaviour, but in his cognitive–behaviour modification approach he stresses the importance of noting the type of self-communication or internal dialogue engaged in *before*, *during*, and *after* the performance of the task (Meichenbaum and Genest, 1982). If one considers the different types of negative thoughts which accompany these three stages in the performance of a task, negative thinking can be systematically tackled and inhibited. Since many dysphonics appear to experience conflict over speaking out, the following is an example of observing negative thoughts and changing them to positive thoughts prior, during, and following an event associated with expressing a personal view:

Negative thoughts	*Positive thoughts*
Before	
I might not get it out perfectly.	I don't have to say it right. Why make it hard for myself by demanding perfection. I'll prepare what I want to say and that will help. I have everything to gain and nothing to lose.
He's not going to like it.	He can't kill me for saying what I think. If I don't say what I think, he'll walk all over me. If I speak my mind our relationship will be more honest. I might even get more respect.
During	
He's not listening.	If he is not listening that's his difficulty. I'll just have to repeat my view.
He's starting to look angry and to raise his voice.	If he is getting angry and and raising his voice it's probably because he is being defensive. I won't let this fluster me and I won't be drawn or provoked into an emotional reaction of anxiety or anger. By staying calm I'll think more rationally. The important thing is to relax.
I can't stand anyone being angry at me.	Of course I can stand it. I might prefer it if people weren't angry with me but it isn't possible always to agree with everyone all the time. I have every right to hold the views I do and every right to express them, just as he does.
After	
I don't think he really understood me.	If he didn't understand me he probably wasn't listening and that's his problem not mine.

I should have said it more clearly. I might want to re-phrase some things I said to make them clearer but I don't think that would make a significant difference. Overall, I said most of what I wanted and that's the important thing. Instead of looking for minor 'failings' and exaggerating them I ought to tell myself how well I did, how much I was in control and also how well I coped in handling difficult moments. What's more, if I can do it once, I can do it again and it should be easier next time.

Diaphragmatic breathing

The negative thinking described in the previous example would probably have had a physical effect, causing such things as increased blood adrenaline, changes in breathing rate and muscular tension. While positive self-instruction may be sufficient to reverse the anxiety response, the physical reactions can have a life of their own and can 'run on' if not checked. Also, rather than relying on positive self-instruction alone, many people find it helpful to have additional strategies which help them gain control over the physical effects of the anxiety reaction. Therefore, after positive self-instruction (which can be as systematic and comprehensive as the above example or as simple as telling oneself to 'relax') has been used, the third step in rapid stress control is to focus on slowing down breathing. This is done by inhaling slowly and by employing diaphragmatic rather than thoracic muscles. Essentially, as one breathes in, one focuses on filling the lungs by pushing out the stomach rather than the chest. The therapist can demonstrate this by putting one hand on his or her own chest, the other at the top of the stomach (where the ribs arch over the belly) and showing how it is mainly the abdomen which moves when one breathes diaphragmatically. When the client's lungs feel full, he or she is asked to hold the breath for a few moments and release the air as slowly as possible. In voice therapy the therapist will ask the client to relax the throat at this point.

The rationale for focusing on the breathing is presented as follows: focusing on breathing is a means of inhibiting any tendency to hyperventilate and can have a valuable psychological affect by helping clients feel that they are taking control as well as slowing themselves down. In addition, patients can be encouraged to associate the release of breath with the release of tension, thus producing a sense of 'letting go', relief and relaxation as they breathe out. As speech pathologists are aware, another important reason for focusing on reducing thoracic breathing with voice patients is that thoracic breathing does not provide adequate breath support for normal voice and creates tension in the throat. Diaphragmatic breathing reverses this pattern and encourages a relaxed vocal tract and good breath support for voice.

Rapid relaxation

The final step in rapid stress control is to employ the skill of rapid physical relaxation. This can be done by utilising the progressive muscular relaxation technique of systematically observing any tension in individual muscles and, beginning with the hands and fingers, arms and legs, simply relaxing the muscles one by one throughout the body (see the description of this procedure in step 12 of *Progressive muscular relaxation*). This is done while the diaphragmatic breath is released and, typically, a person will get about half way through the relaxation before needing to take a second breath. As the second breath is released, he or she should focus on relaxing muscles in the lower half of the body. The procedure can be illustrated by the simile of passing a spotlight of consciousness stage by stage over the whole body. Most people report that with practice the whole procedure becomes condensed, so that on taking a slow, diaphragmatic breath they simply, and more or less instantaneously, relax the whole of their body. However, even when the technique is being learnt, relaxation is very rapid and will be completed in a space of two deep breaths or about 30 seconds.

Not only is the whole procedure of rapid stress control quick but it cannot be observed by others. Thus it can be practised in any situation without self-consciousness. If going through rapid stress control once does not reduce anxiety difficulties or if the effects are not long lasting, the procedure can be repeated until the desired results are achieved. If on completion, however, a person wants to repeat it immediately, we advise that he or she take a less exaggerated diaphragmatic breath initially or make sure they breathe out very slowly in order to avoid any possibility of causing light-headedness etc.

By using rapid stress control as a foundation for anxiety and stress management, the clinician can complement this widely applicable approach with a variety of cognitive–behavioural strategies. An appropriate choice of strategies will arise from the initial and ongoing assessment of the individual case. The following sections and case examples should illustrate this point.

Life stresses

As was mentioned in Chapter 3, research has indicated that anxiety and depression, as well as physical illness, often follow one or more major life events or a series of minor life events. In working with psychogenic dysphonia we have noted the presence of stressful life events such as the following: a spouse's unemployment, increases in personal responsibilities, life role changes, more demanding work etc., a move from a family environment, changes in and concerns about a child's behaviour, a decline in health or the protracted or terminal illness of a close relative, and bereavement. Furthermore, the development of aphonia or dysphonia at these times creates an additional stress since the person feels more vulnerable or 'fragile' and may suffer from lowered self-confidence. The loss of voice requires adaptation and often makes carrying out most professions quite difficult.

A number of strategies within a cognitive–behavioural framework can be employed as a response to helping the person cope with these life events. For example, initial input would probably be *educational* in the sense of providing information about life events (see Chapter 3, *The influence of recent life events*, p.46) and the symptoms caused by stress. Many patients fail to acknowledge just how stressful their life has been, particularly when life changes fall within a range usually considered quite minor. When asked to review the changes which have occurred in the past year, patients are often surprised at the number of adjustments they have had to make over a relatively short period of time. Many find it helpful to recognise that, in the context of all these changes, they have a right to be anxious or stressed.

Spending time helping people consider how they can reduce additional stress will usually produce valuable results. For example, where people are thinking of changing occupations in order to reduce stress, they should first be asked to consider what new demands they might expect to take on which could prove to be as stressful or more stressful then their current situation. They should then be asked to consider whether there are changes they could make in their current job which might not only reduce stress but also give them a sense of control. When people complain that their jobs are too stressful, one strategy can be to challenge them with what they are going to do about changing these stresses – thus placing responsibility directly on their own shoulders – and then guiding and supporting them in finding solutions.

Reducing and ending the habit of worry

Since in many cases the anxiety caused by worrying reduces problem-solving capacities, anxious, excessive worriers may find it helpful to be told that they are only allowed to worry during a set half-hour a day (Borkovec et al., 1983). If they catch themselves worrying at other times, they must put this off until it is time to give their full attention to solving their difficulties. The value of a technique like this can be illustrated by the case of a school teacher who complained that his roster and the demands of difficult children were so stressful that he could no longer cope. On being encouraged to take more responsibility for the situation, to look for ways of gaining control, rather than being controlled by the school system, and to use a daily half-hour problem-solving strategy as a means of doing this, he quickly found a solution. This involved approaching his deputy head to suggest that the timetable be changed and that problem children be distributed to other classes. When the changes were carried out, they considerably altered daily pressures and were a major factor in reducing the teacher's anxiety (Butcher, 1984).

Patients who worry excessively can also be trained to question the nature of their worries in terms of whether these are productive or unproductive worries. For example, one dysphonic patient, having been given guidance on self-observation and 'thought catching', noted that she had a tendency to take her worries home from work. To counter this tendency she was encouraged to question the value of this pursuit and asked to consider whether the worries were productive or unproductive worries. It was explained that productive worries are the sort that if you spend some time thinking about a difficulty you will find a solution, while unproductive worries are those that, no matter how much you worry, nothing will change. (For example, worrying about being burgled can be productive if you then improve the security of your home but unproductive if you then continue to worry when nothing more can be done.) On looking at her worries in this way, the patient noted that many of her worries were of the unproductive sort. At this point she was instructed on how to deal with these thoughts by using a single strategy: whenever she noticed that she was caught up in unproductive thoughts she was asked to disrupt them by using diaphragmatic breathing and rapid relaxation to 'get out of her head into her body' and then to disrupt the thoughts further and distract herself by becoming involved in an external (preferably physical or non-passive) activity. When implemented, this procedure proved to be an important means of stress reduction. As a way of introducing this strategy, we have often found it helpful to cite the Gestalt therapist Barry Stevens:

> The more that I observe, the more that I see the process of thinking, the easier it is for me to let my fantasies go. When I am not observing them, they possess me ...I don't mean that there's nothing to worry about. There are *always* lots and lots of things to worry about. It's just that there's no point or usefulness in worrying about them. My observation is that either what I worry about doesn't happen – or it happens anyway. All that my worrying has accomplished is to make me miserable.

(Stevens, 1977, p.196-197)

While patients experiencing stressful life events will benefit from supportive counselling or having the opportunity to talk about their feelings, the use of more confrontational and directive cognitive–behavioural strategies by the therapist can be beneficial. For example, from a cognitive point of view, if a woman is saying of her husband's unemployment that 'nothing ever goes right and he will never get a job again', the therapist may ask her to question these thoughts as follows: 'It's hard to imagine that nothing has ever gone right in your life! Can you recall things that have turned out well? Perhaps you can think of times when things looked as black as this and you got over them? ... Perhaps you have a tendency to expect things always to go smoothly when really the world is not like that? ... Maybe you are saying it *must* go smoothly or you can't cope? If so, perhaps you need to question these thoughts, to remind yourself of when you coped before and got through difficult times, to tell yourself that, while it may be difficult, you have resources you can draw on which will help you through it ... You can't say for certain that your husband will never get a job. It may be difficult now but things could change. Worrying and getting anxious won't help and even if the situation doesn't change, perhaps we can spend some time exploring helpful ways of looking at this, perhaps looking at things you can do which will help you adapt to this situation ... etc.'

The cognitive approach can be adapted to other stresses and losses (such as worrying over a relative's declining health) and even to bereavement counselling provided it is done sensitively. In some of these cases this leads on to issues surrounding feelings of guilt – the patient feeling they should do more for the person they are concerned about or should have done more for the person they have lost. The therapist can question how rational these thoughts are (we have more to say on this later in this chapter) and sometimes there will be specific behavioural strategies which are helpful. For example, with one dysphonic who was deeply distressed by a feud in her family which kept her from seeing her terminally ill sister, a good deal of stress was taken off her shoulders by the speech pathologist suggesting that she express her thoughts and feelings in a letter, which was then sent to her sister.

Common difficulties with family and interpersonal relationships

The most common life stresses found in association with psychogenic voice disorder have been noted to be interpersonal relationship difficulties, anxieties surrounding the expression of opinions or views (conflict over speaking out), overcommitment or taking the onus of responsibility, and feelings of powerlessness concerning any ability to make positive change. Usually these difficulties are closely interrelated. For example, a common reason why interpersonal difficulties exist is that a person has failed to assert his or her views. Similarly, some individuals assume the burden of responsibility in the family because they lack the appropriate assertiveness skills to set limits and/or to resist coercion. Certainly, a high proportion of dysphonics are embroiled in unhappy relationships of one sort or another. Commonly their relationships with their partners are poor and many of the females in this group are married to men who are insensitive to their needs. The poor communication within the marriage and general difficulties often extend to conflicts with their children but are also observable in the presence of wider family disruptions. For example, a major cause of stress for one dysphonic was discovering that while she was in hospital following a miscarriage, her husband had an affair with her immature, manipulative sister, who she also knew was planning to move to a house opposite their own. Examples such as this may explain why Aronson et al. (1966) found that a high percentage of dysphonics report confusion and insecurity around sexuality.

Given the high incidence of marital discord, therapy will frequently be concerned with this issue. Most cognitive–behaviour therapists would prefer to see both partners together or, where there are difficulties with other family members, to get them personally involved in treatment. In practice, this usually proves difficult as spouses, teenage children and other family members are often unwilling and sometimes unable to attend. Thus, we usually find that, although we have encouraged the patient to bring a family member along to sessions, we are forced to work independently with the patient in order to bring about change.

While each case must be treated as unique and as having individual needs, the common themes in treating marital and family discord will be *improving communication, increasing problem-solving skills and the rewards of marriage,* and *training in assertiveness* (especially speaking out) or *setting limits with others.*

Communication

Since good communication is at the very least a two-way affair (a message has to be received and understood as well as sent), the therapist is at a disadvantage when working with just one person from a family where communication is poor. However, through role playing the therapist can illustrate helpful and unhelpful forms of communication, as well as provide the patient with practice, feedback and an appropriate model of how to deal with specific issues. The basic strategy is to explore an area where a person is finding communication difficult and then for the therapist to play the role of the spouse, daughter, etc. as the difficult exchange is rehearsed. The therapist will need to know something about the role to be played and will need to ask such things as 'How do you think your husband would react if you said ...?', 'Do you think he is the sort of person who would ...?', 'What do you think you daughter would say if you said it this way...?'. Once into the role playing, it is usually easy to demonstrate the alternative consequences of expressing things in different ways. The therapist can then make observations about how the patient expresses views and how this makes the recipient feel, as well as giving feedback on what needs to be changed in order to reduce such things as defensive reactions or mis-understanding. Reversing roles, so that, for example, the patient plays her husband and the therapist the patient, can help the patient experi-ence how the other might feel or react differently when the same issue is presented in different ways. Here such simple behavioural strategies as learning to give praise before criticism can reduce the chances of a defensive reaction. The difference can be seen in the following two exchanges:

Wife: (feeling exasperated) I never see you these days. You never do anything for me any more. You never help me out or help out with the kids.

Husband: (losing his temper) Don't you think I'm tired when I get in?! Do you think you're the only one working a long day? What makes you so perfect? Anyway, who'd want to come home to someone who's always complaining?

Wife: You know, I really appreciate how hard you are working these days – all those long hours – it really helps financially – but I do miss your company and so do the kids. When you used to spend time with them it used to give me a break as well. I'm wondering if the extra money is worth it, particularly when it's making you so tired?

Husband: I thought you wanted the over-time for extra things around the house, but maybe you're right, maybe we'd all be hap-pier if I did less hours.

Increasing problem-solving skills and rewards

Improving communication skills should make the marriage a more rewarding experience for both husband and wife. In those situations where both partners have agreed to enter therapy, many therapists focus on helping them improve their problem-solving skills and the rewards of marriage. Since, by definition, a problem is intrinsically unrewarding, it can be safely assumed that eliminating a problem will usually increase marital rewards. One way of solving problems and making a marriage more rewarding is to compile a list of complaints which each partner makes about the other and then to use this list to look for problem solutions or ways of reaching an acceptable compromise. Further to this, change can often be achieved through the partners agreeing on a *mutual exchange of rewards*. For example, if the husband's list contains a complaint that his wife cooks too many processed meals and his wife retorts that she cooks quick meals because she rarely has enough time to prepare something more elaborate, he might agree to be more helpful with the children and household chores in exchange for more 'home cooking'. Thus, while both have to 'earn' their rewards (he by helping in the home and she by giving the time to prepare the meals), they both gain things which are important to them in terms of making their marriage more rewarding.

Assertiveness and setting limits with others

When it comes to assertiveness and setting limits with others, role playing can be a helpful way of allowing the patient to rehearse what needs to be said and to practise a combination of cognitive and behavioural strategies. In many situations, looking at thoughts before, during and after practising being assertive (as illustrated earlier on in this chapter, pages 84–86) can be very helpful. This enables people to begin dealing with self-defeating thoughts and to start encouraging themselves in what they are trying to do.

The following two case examples will illustrate some interpersonal difficulties and treatment approaches used in the presence of difficulties in assertiveness.

Doris, a 45-year-old patient who, during the past 23 years, had suffered five periods of aphonia, had a long history of difficulty in expressing her thoughts and emotions. She was of the view that if she expressed what she felt she would probably 'go to pieces'. During treatment she was initially asked to keep a record of those times when she found it difficult to voice her views ; her first focus was on how to respond appropriately to an acquaintance who called more frequently than she wished and who often came at an inconvenient time. Even after the psychologist and speech pathologist had role-played the situation for her in order to provide a model of how to express her views, Doris was so inhibited that she could not practise this in role playing. However, during the following week, she was able to say something to her visitor which implied that it might be an inconvenient time to call as she was planning to go out. Unfortunately, the visitor did not take the hint. Having praised Doris for attempting to take control of the situation, the therapist suggested that she might take what she had done a step further by continuing to get ready to leave her home and physically showing her visitor that she was going out. In following this advice the next time her visitor called, Doris also found the courage to say that the frequent visits were unwelcome and, thereafter, her friend called less often. When followed up six months after her discharge, Doris was coping extremely well, despite a number of life stresses during this time – including a hysterectomy – and had not experienced any voice loss. She reported being much more able to be assertive and to express her views and it was clear that she no longer feared 'going to pieces' if she did so.

Maureen, aged 49, was born into a large Irish family of 17 children and had married at the age of 20 a rather unassertive man; they had lived in England for most of their married life. They had five children, who were then aged between 21 and 28 years. She felt she had failed as a mother or 'went wrong with all of the children' and that they were all 'head-strong'. Two of her sons had been involved with drugs and, when she was seen, one son was in prison for stealing.

Maureen presented in the ENT Department with a six-month history of dysphonia and was referred for speech therapy following the removal of a nodule from her vocal cord. She was seen for a brief course of voice therapy before a further admission to remove a nodule from the other vocal cord. Thereafter, she was seen for further voice therapy without significant benefit. During this period, the therapist noted that, among other psychological factors associated with her dysphonia, Maureen had 'great difficulty in expressing her feelings' and that she admitted bottling up a lot of feelings inside herself. This was particularly the case in relation to her sister-in-law, who lived nearby, visited frequently and whom she felt interfered with her life and manipulated both her husband and herself. Maureen felt unable to stand up to her sister-in-law's coercion and felt unexpressed anger toward her. When Maureen was referred at this stage to a psychologist for an opinion, the psychologist's assessment also supported the view that Maureen's difficulty asserting herself with her sister-in-law was currently the major cause of ongoing stress and had probably precipitated and was maintaining her voice loss. At this time it was also noted that Maureen had difficulty expressing her views to authority figures in her work as a cleaner in a home for the elderly. Her lack of assertiveness in this area was considered to be a further source of stress. In addition, the previous week her youngest daughter had left a note saying that she had gone to live with her boyfriend but did not say where; this was considered to be another, current, source of stress.

After the psychologist's assessment it was arranged that Maureen would be seen jointly and should be taught anxiety management and rapid stress control techniques in addition to the relaxation she had learnt in speech and language therapy. For the next week she was asked to keep a record of all stressful interactions with her sister-in-law and any thoughts and feelings which accompanied these occasions.

Maureen found it difficult to write down her thoughts and feelings during the week but, by focusing at the following session on what she would like to say to her sister-in-law, she was able to say that she was mainly inhibited in speaking her mind by the fear of overreacting, going too far or being too cruel, hurting her sister-in-law and creating a situation wherein they would end up not speaking. After discussing her fears and briefly considering how to speak her mind, in the following week Maureen was able to resist her sister-in-law's coercion over something she wanted to do in her own way and to assert herself appropriately without any of the disastrous consequences she had previously predicted.

During the following three weeks, other worries came to the fore, including worries caused by discovering that her runaway daughter was pregnant and worries about her own physical health because of severe pains in the side. During therapy she was reassured that she was taking a sensible attitude to her daughter's predicament – providing the right level of support without interfering or making decisions for her – and had taken the appropriate steps to put her mind at rest about her physical health by going to the local hospital for a medical check-up. Without prompting, she said that she had concluded that her physical pains were stress-related: 'All these worries tie my guts in knots'. Despite these additional challenges, Maureen had continued to speak her mind and to resist coercion from her sister-in-law and had been more direct and outspoken with her husband over domestic and family matters. The third session focused on her inability to accompany her husband to a regular quiz night at his social club. Her refusal to attend led her husband to complain that they no longer socialised together. Assessment showed that she was afraid to accept his invitation to join him out of a fear of not being able to answer the questions and of making a fool of herself. Her avoidance was tackled both cognitively and behaviourally by helping her find positive thoughts to defeat her fears and then by asking her to target accepting her husband's invitation in the following week. When seen two weeks later, she had been able to attend the quiz night and gave examples of being assertive with various people. Her success not only pleased her but also pleased her husband, who felt she was making some effort in their marriage. She had continued to get the pains in her side but these had been less frequent. She was still worried about her daughter, but when she telephoned, Maureen had been firm with her. Maureen felt satisfied with this, since she felt it was the right response. She was particularly pleased about her progress in speaking her mind and said she felt she was no longer 'a mouse'.

Maureen's voice had continued to improve over this period but, following an altercation at the home for the elderly when Maureen felt she was being treated unjustly and defended herself vigorously, she lost her voice for two days. A week later, in the therapy session, it was still not as good as it had been at her previous appointment. During this session the focus was on the way assertiveness can sometimes have negative consequences when it does not go exactly to plan or when the other person becomes belligerent or defensive, but there was also a focus on reassuring her that her progress had been genuine and on reminding her of all she had achieved. In particular, it was stressed that it was important for her not to lose sight of the gains, not to exaggerate the difficulties and not to distort the consequences (i.e. the voice loss) into failure when, in fact, she had not failed in her most important target of being more assertive.

At this point in treatment Maureen took a holiday in Ireland and for a number of reasons was unable to attend appointments immediately on her return, so that she was not seen for three months. However, she had maintained her progress. Overall, her voice was now very good and on some days returned to normal. Moreover, she said that she was now more aware of the way her emotional state affected voice quality. Since the therapists noticed a tendency to strain when initiating voice, the speech pathologist suggested making an individual appointment to begin working on disrupting this habit. When followed up over the next four months, Maureen continued to maintain her assertiveness (she was clearly doing this appropriately since she said she and her sister-in-law were now 'the best of friends') and, although this was sometimes at the cost of losing her voice for short periods (particularly after asserting herself at work), overall her voice remained much improved, her anxiety state was significantly reduced and she reported being much happier with her quality of life.

The difficult adolescent

In those cases where children create interpersonal stress, it is not uncommon to find that the relationship is unhealthy because of parental overinvolvement or mother–child separation difficulties and the inability on the part of a parent to gain appropriate control or set adequate limits. For example, one patient, Iris, complained that her main source of tension grew out of an extremely difficult relationship with her 18-year-old daughter, Tina. Psychological assessment suggested that a number of factors made the relationship pathological. At heart, mother and daughter were extremely attached and dependent on each other and one thing Iris feared was that, if she upset her daughter, Tina would leave home and their relationship would be destroyed. Because of this fear, Iris found it difficult to set limits or to be strict with her daughter and usually gave in to her demands. Furthermore, from a very early age, whenever she was punished Tina had developed the strategy of having a tantrum and then withdrawing her love or rejecting Iris through long periods of silence and critical looks. Iris found this withdrawal of love deeply distressing and always gave into Tina in order to be reassured that she had not destroyed her daughter's love for her. Because of this pattern, Iris saw her daughter as very powerful, someone who always went her own way, established independence and could never be punished. In this context Iris described herself and her daughter as opposites; she was soft, warm and loving, while Tina was hard, cold, independent and hurting. Her daughter's independence, however, was very superficial and she often became very attention seeking. For example, when Iris was in hospital Tina deliberately put her hand through a pane of glass in what was thought to be an attempt to get more attention. She could also be very violent and out of control in response to what would normally be considered reasonable requests from her mother. Thus, for Iris, a central concern was how to retain control over her daughter.

Following the assessment and detailed analysis of the pattern of disagreement, an initial contract of six sessions was offered to Iris in which she agreed to the following aims: first, to see if she could view the relationship from a different viewpoint and to see if she could develop more insight into the neurotic or destructive pattern which existed between her and her daughter; second, to try a new approach when dealing with Tina's tantrums, her withdrawal of love, silence and critical looks, by *making her own love a condition of acceptable behaviour*. This would be done by telling Tina to go to her room if she wanted to have a tantrum, encouraging her to act in a more mature way or to take 'grown-up' responsibilities and, most importantly of all, if Tina continued to sulk, Iris would 'turn the tables' on the withdrawal of love and the silent criticism by saying that she would not forgive Tina's childish behaviour *unless* there was a clear demonstration that she could be better behaved.

This programme was set up a few days after an incident when Tina attacked Iris with a hairbrush. Over the coming weeks Iris was consistently able to remind Tina that behaving in this way was completely unacceptable and that she would not forgive her daughter unless she demonstrated a change in her behaviour. Although Tina initially responded in her usual way, Iris remained firm and did not give into her fear of driving her daughter away. Then, although it took some weeks and there were a number of testing moments, Tina's behaviour changed dramatically from being selfish, disobedient and frequently uncontrolled or violent, to being obedient, helpful and even sharing her concerns about important life decisions in a more mature way. On review a year later, Iris had coped well with Tina getting a boyfriend, their first major separation when Tina went on holiday and the news that she planned to move into her own flat. During that year Tina's behaviour had generally been more acceptable, but there had been three occasions when she reverted to her old behaviour. On each occasion Iris remained firm, said clearly to Tina that if she was going to behave like that she, Iris, did not like her daughter's attitude nor like her as a person and would not change her views without a demonstration from Tina that she could behave in a mature and acceptable manner. As a consequence the relapses were short lived and the stresses in Iris's life much less than when she was seen initially. Iris consistently regained her normal voice shortly after initiating the changes outlined above and experienced no loss of voice throughout the year over which she was followed up.

Programmes of this sort are based on principles of operant conditioning, which show that, as a general rule, behaviour which is rewarded or reinforced will increase in frequency and behaviour which is not reinforced will decline in frequency (Karoly, 1982). The following case provides a further example of how operant conditioning principles can be applied in treatment.

Helen, who was a 41-year-old dysphonic, complained of family difficulties. Her relationship with her husband was said to be poor. He was uncommunicative and the poor relationship was made worse by the fact that they were both working and employed on different shifts, so that they rarely saw each other. Helen was especially perturbed by the fact that her husband failed to take enough responsibility in the family and did not support her efforts to get their children to be helpful. She worked an extremely long day, both before and after her work shifts, and was particularly at odds with her slothful 18-year-old daughter, Penny, whom she described as 'untidy', 'lazy' and 'disobedient'. For example, Penny would discard clothes in the living room and not pick them up when asked. Penny's behaviour made Helen resentful but she said she found it difficult to keep telling her daughter to do things out of a fear of 'making her in my own image', by which she meant making Penny into a person like herself, who was always having to do things for others.

Along with a focus on the communication difficulties in her relationship with her husband and helping her to question critically the reality of her fear of making her daughter 'a Cinderella', at the first session Helen was given the homework task of making a list of chores she would like to be carried out by Penny. At the second session she brought along a list of eight changes she would like Penny to make. After considering various strategies, Helen agreed to approach her daughter with a contract as follows: Penny would be asked to carry out a chore and would be reminded a short time later if it had not been done, but if at that stage Penny did not comply and Helen had to do it, Penny would be 'charged for this service'. The agreed rate was 25p (50c) for each 'item'. This 'service charge' was to be deducted from Penny's weekly pocket money. All charges would be recorded as promptly as possible to ensure an accurate record of debits. Penny was also informed that if all her pocket money was used up for the coming week, further charges would be debited from the pocket money she should receive for the following week, and so on.

The therapist made a point of warning Helen that the plan might not go smoothly. It is common with programmes of this sort to make adjustments to details (for example, the amount charged might need to be different in order to balance her pocket money with the number of chores which are typical within a week). Just as commonly, the individual whose behaviour is being changed will not comply initially, either because they test out the system in order to see if the person they are in conflict with actually means what they say or to see if they can still get away with their old behaviour. For this latter reason, the therapist also stressed the importance of Helen not wavering in her resolve to carry out what she had agreed with him and, more importantly, had agreed with her daughter. However, in this case there were no major problems with, or changes to, the plan. There was an immediate positive response from Penny and, as a consequence, Helen reported not only that she felt more relaxed at home but also generally that Penny was easier to live with and was much more helpful. However, there was no major improvement in Helen's voice. Since the other stresses remained the same, it was assumed that the change in her relationship with her daughter was too minor to have a significant effect. Unfortunately, Helen dropped out of treatment before the therapists could focus on any further means of stress reduction.

The difficult parent

Another source of family stress for many patients comes from an overly demanding or controlling elderly parent. For one patient, Evelyne, with an eight-to-nine-year history of hoarseness and dysphonia, the main source of stress was caring for her 90-year-old mother, who lived with Evelyne and her husband in a small apartment. Assessment suggested that Evelyne's mother had always been demanding and difficult, constantly complaining, expecting things to be done for her and making little or no effort to help herself or her daughter. Evelyne admitted to being too caring, giving her mother too much attention and spoiling her in the past. More recently, her mother had shown evidence of Alzheimer's disease and her forgetfulness had been a particular strain. Unfortunately, given the deterioration in Evelyne's mother, it was not feasible to offer a great deal through cognitive–behaviour therapy other than acknowledging the strain Evelyne was coping with (and through this reinforcing her strengths) and suggesting the behavioural strategy of getting additional breaks from her mother by going out of the apartment more frequently.

In other cases, it has been possible to suggest more. For example, where a daughter has taken the sole responsibility for caring for a difficult, elderly mother, we have not only focused on the cognitive strategy of helping her question the guilty feelings of not doing enough, but on questioning whether the parent is her responsibility alone or whether there are others who can help, questioning whether the more she does the less the parent will try to help and whether this is good for the parent's self-esteem, etc. In helping the patient reframe her situation and her obligations, it is also possible to guide her in setting behavioural targets. These can, for instance, include asking another family member for help, setting the parent small challenges and rewarding the parent's efforts with encouragement and praise, finding out about social services, meals-on-wheels, etc., experimenting with reducing the frequency of visits (one patient made a detour every day to and from work in order to see her mother and to do chores) and so on.

Feelings of powerlessness

As can be seen from the above examples, the strategies employed by the therapist can help patients make changes which alter their situations and the stresses involved in their being overinvolved, overcommitted, unable to set limits or unable to speak out. As will be appreciated, situations of this sort engender feelings of powerlessness. Extensive research has indicated that loss of control or no longer feeling personally effective in relationships or situations is extremely stressful for individuals (Rotter, 1966; Seligman, 1975; Bandura, 1989) and can create both depressive and anxiety disorders. Thus, we take the view that consideration of ways to enhance the individual sense of personal efficacy will often be an important element in cognitive–behaviour therapy. The following strategies can be seen as means to achieve a sense of being personally effective or in control: role playing or rehearsal; considering and implementing targets; learning new skills (such as positive self-statements, ending negative or worrying thoughts and rapid stress control); speaking out; assertive actions (such as setting limits or initiating a behavioural reinforcement programme); observing that it is possible to create change and to improve a difficult or intolerable situation; and generally getting feedback from events and from others that control is not only a possibility but a reality which can be grasped.

Whilst there are other cognitive–behavioural methods which we found were helpful in responding to individual cases of psychogenic dysphonia, such approaches (including systematic desensitisation and strategies to improve decision making skills and time use) were in the minority and, whilst there may be individual differences which require treatment strategies not discussed, we hope to have illustrated some of the more common themes or difficulties and how these can be construed and treated. Those wishing to develop additional knowledge of cognitive–behavioural strategies would benefit from consulting Kanfer and Goldstein (1982) and Hawton et al. (1989), which, from their slightly different perspectives, provide a fairly comprehensive description of strategies.

A case study

We conclude this chapter with a detailed case study. This charts the development of psychogenic dysphonia in the context of life stresses and a depressive-anxiety reaction, illustrates some of the common issues which have to be addressed with this population and shows many of the strategies which can be employed in treatment.

Background information and formulation

Sharon, aged 25, was originally referred to a psychologist because she had consulted her general practitioner, complaining of feeling depressed and having agoraphobic symptoms. She was the younger of two children and described having a good relationship with her parents and her elder brother. Sharon had done reasonably well at school but could probably have done better if she had not been obsessed with dancing and had not neglected her school work. She said that dancing was the only thing she had ever really wanted to do. When she left school she became a professional dancer, but stopped when she became pregnant at the age of 21. Sharon had been in a long-term relationship with the father of her child but had recently discovered that he was also having a relationship with one of her friends. He left her when she was three-months pregnant. Following the birth of her daughter, Nicola, Sharon lost her confidence in herself as a dancer and was unable to return to this career. However, for a while she had some success as a model. Eventually, however, work became so infrequent that she was forced to take less and less glamorous employment, working at an airport desk, then in a shop selling clothes and, most recently, collecting the takings from gambling machines. She felt that the loss of a career as either a dancer or a model was significant in causing a loss of self-confidence. In relation to this, the first interview elicited an important schema in her thinking when she revealed: 'All my life I had to be better than the girl next door'. It was probably this desire for excellence that led to a period of anorexia at the age of 18 when she was developing her career as a dancer. Since the birth of her daughter she had had one relationship of five months, which did not work out and for the past two years she had been in a relationship with a man, Kevin, whom she planned to marry in six months time.

Assessment of specific events precipitating her symptoms of anxiety and depression suggested that these began shortly after she lost her job at the airport and when she was having difficulties with the manager in her new job as an assistant in a clothing store. It was assumed that the loss of a more glamorous career, the defeat of her ambitions in someone who always had to be better than others, the difficulties with her boss when adapting to a new job and the decline in self-confidence were all important precipitating factors. Since that time she had experienced frequent bouts of tearfulness and panic attacks involving sweating, shaking, breathing difficulties, dizziness and pins and needles in hands and fingers. She was usually anxious in crowds and when using public transport, but was better when with company and normally had no difficulty when driving herself.

When she lost her job at the airport, her wedding to her fiancé, Kevin, had to be called off for financial reasons. However, ambivalence about the impending marriage and difficulty expressing her views seemed to be two other important causes of her depressive/anxiety state. Whilst there were good things in the relationship with Kevin, in that she felt he genuinely loved both herself and her daughter, did a great deal for them and tried to boost her confidence by encouraging her to keep trying with modelling, on the negative side she felt that he ruled her life. She did not feel that he gave her any opportunity in most situations to say what she wanted to do and she stressed that 'he treats me like a little girl'.

Treatment

At the conclusion of the first session, Sharon was offered a course of treatment beginning with learning anxiety management via the pre-recorded audio tape described above and was asked to keep a daily record of situations which elicited worrying thoughts. Over the first three sessions therapy was focused largely on helping Sharon master diaphragmatic breathing and improving the communication and the rewards in her relationship with Kevin. These sessions explored how she might be more outspoken about her feelings and she was able to put some of this into practice. However, when seen the following week, she had developed a dysphonic condition and could only speak in a hoarse whisper! Whilst there was every reason to assume that this was psychogenic, arrangements were made for her to have an ENT assessment. However, her voice returned to normal shortly before the consultation and she cancelled this appointment.

The day before Sharon lost her voice, Kevin's mother had given her a wedding bouquet which she did not like, but she felt unable to say so through fear of offending her future mother-in-law. The following day Sharon's dog chewed up the bouquet and Sharon did not have the courage to inform Kevin's mother. It was on this day that she lost her voice. At this session Sharon admitted that although she had been more frank with Kevin about a number of concerns relating to the forthcoming marriage, there were also 'lots of things I haven't been able to say to Kevin'. As a consequence of discussing more fully her difficulty in speaking her mind, she agreed to invite Kevin along to the next session so that the therapist could help her take the step of being more honest with her partner.

When Kevin attended the next meeting the impression he gave was of someone with a forceful personality and it was noticeable that he tended to take charge of the session. Whilst observing them relate to each other showed that there was a lot of warmth, humour and love in the relationship, it was also easy to see why Sharon saw Kevin as controlling. When Kevin was informed by the therapist of Sharon's conflict over speaking out, he countered that he felt that he also could not speak his mind because if he did Sharon overreacted. Sharon replied strongly that although this might be true currently, she never used to be like that. Their difficulty in communicating was then highlighted by Sharon giving an example of where she felt he was controlling and had belittled her in front of his friends. Until then she had not been able to discuss the incident but had seethed inside. They had been discussing the wedding plans with two friends and Sharon had mentioned that on the day she planned to have her make-up done professionally. Kevin had told her in no uncertain terms that she was not to get it done professionally, but should do it herself. During the session, Kevin justified his comments by explaining that this was meant as a compliment since he believed that she could do it better herself. However, he had the good grace to admit that, like his mother, he tended to be bossy and blunt, not good at explaining himself and that on this occasion, 'it came out wrong'.

During the session, the therapist was able to emphasise the importance of improving the communication and rewards in the relationship and targets were agreed for the coming week. Since Kevin tended to work long hours, one target, designed to increase the rewards in the relationship, was that he try to set limits with his job in order for them to have more time together. Although Kevin was given an open invitation to attend future sessions, Sharon came alone to subsequent meetings.

At the next session Sharon reported that the last meeting had been helpful and that Kevin was making more effort with communication and in setting limits with his work. She had even spoken her mind over an incident when he expected her to make and bring him a cup of tea first thing in the morning while he lay in bed. However, she experienced one particular conflict over speaking out when, after she had spent some time tidying their home, he came in and made it untidy almost immediately. She had never confronted him about his untidiness and his tendency to expect her to tidy up after him. On this occasion, she said she had not mentioned her annoyance because things had improved and she feared her comments might cause an argument. During the week, however, Sharon's main concern had been with her three-year old daughter, Nicola, who had been very disobedient and oppositional. Thus the session also focused on developing a simple behavioural programme designed to reinforce good behaviour and – with appropriate warning – to remove treats or rewards for undesirable behaviour. The programme was also to include Kevin's cooperation since Sharon felt that he left all the disciplining of Nicola to her.

At the next meeting Sharon reported that she had spoken to Kevin about helping in disciplining Nicola and she was very positive about the effort he had made following her request. However, at this session and over the following weeks Sharon was able to talk in more depth about her fears of marrying Kevin. First, she highlighted how his bossiness was very similar to that of his mother and how she feared that the marriage would give his mother greater influence over her and make her feel more trapped and powerless. Second, she had real conflicts with Kevin over financial matters. When she was short of money he would promise her cash and then fail to provide it. At other times he would borrow money and not repay it. The situation created another conflict for Sharon over speaking out, since she found that if she mentioned these money matters Kevin became angry and this created a scene which usually left a bad atmosphere for days.

Sharon was encouraged to adopt a number of positive cognitive–behavioural strategies in response to these difficulties. First, she could tell herself that there were things she could do to be in control of her situation. One aspect of this would be to continue reminding Kevin what he was doing to her whenever he behaved in a way she construed as 'bossy'. To help her to be less upset by his behaviour and to help her speak out, she should tell herself two things: 'The bossiness is probably a bad habit learnt from his mother and is comprised mainly of putting a request badly' (i.e. ordering rather than asking, telling rather than suggesting or inviting) and also that 'there has been proof in the past weeks that he does change when reminded'. Second, she should ask him to sit down to discuss their financial arrangements and different ways in which they could be organised.

Two weeks later, four weeks prior to the wedding, Sharon had been able to achieve her targets and this had produced some positive results. Furthermore, without setting this as a target, when Kevin continued to be untidy she had pointed out that he was being unfair and, since then, he had been more considerate. She had also become more outspoken in other areas. Following the serious discussion about their financial arrangements, which was generally fruitful, she still felt he was not recognising that there had been a lot of extra bills in recent weeks and he was leaving their payment to her. As a consequence, she returned to the topic of sharing the finances and threatened to call off the wedding if he did not stop taking her for granted and if he did not 'show he is a partner'.

Whilst she was clearly being more assertive, Sharon was having to cope with new stresses in the form of her work becoming more demanding and Nicola's behaviour suddenly becoming very destructive (tearing wallpaper and cutting the heads of flowers). Since Sharon and Kevin were now adopting a consistent, appropriate response to Nicola's bad behaviour, it was assumed that her disobedience and sudden destructiveness could be attributed to one or a combination of the following factors: being spoilt when visiting her father at weekends; being sensitive to the atmosphere surrounding the wedding; seeking attention; and testing her mother's affection. Sharon had already taken the step of stopping the weekend visits and was therefore simply encouraged to keep up her consistent response of not reinforcing Nicola's unwanted behaviour. Because she had been neglecting to practice the rapid stress control techniques, she was asked to go back to basics and to target listening to the tape more frequently.

The following week, Sharon reported that Nicola's behaviour had improved and that she had been able to carry out her stress management training much more regularly. However, she had found herself in another dilemma over speaking out when a mutual friend of Kevin's mother revealed that her future mother-in-law did not believe that Sharon's dog had chewed up the bouquet and implied that it was just an excuse because Sharon did not like it. Sharon's dilemma was that she could not say anything because, if she did, she would have to reveal that their mutual friend had not kept a confidence and this would cause trouble among all three.

At this session Sharon also reported that, while Kevin had continued to be much more tidy and was consistently less bossy, he was still not working with her 'as a partner' over financial matters. She was having difficulty paying her bills and he was not helping. It was agreed that he needed to be confronted again over this matter. The therapist highlighted once more how she had evidence that speaking her mind to Kevin had worked well so far, with problems over tidiness, bossiness and disciplining Nicola, and that he did change when pressed or when reminded if he had slipped back into old habits.

When seen two weeks later, the day before the wedding, Sharon reported that she was feeling very tense and had been having frequent attacks of panic during recent days. She admitted that two weeks earlier she had felt that she could not go through with the wedding. However, among the changes she had been able to make during those two weeks she had been able to speak to Kevin again about helping with the bills and had done something else which she felt very pleased about. Following a misunderstanding with Kevin's sister about a year previously, there had been considerable tension between her and Sharon throughout that time and the issue had never been properly aired. Until then Sharon had been unable to broach the subject, but, being determined that her wedding day would not be spoilt by family tensions, she visited Kevin's sister and spoke to her about the matter, resolving the misunderstanding and clearing the air. She said that this was a great relief, as was knowing that the wedding preparations were completed. She also felt confident that she could now make the marriage work.

Outcome

Since the beginning of her dysphonia, Sharon's voice had remained a just audible, often hoarse, whisper. On the day before the wedding and for the first time in three months there was a noticeable improvement in volume and quality. When asked about her voice during the previous week, she replied that it had been exactly the same until that day when 'it's the strongest it's been.' She added that 'it feels as though it is going to burst out at any minute.' A little later she also spontaneously commented on how not being able to speak had often given her an excuse to opt out of conflicts, thus giving a clear example of one of the gains associated with voice loss. However, it was 3–4 weeks before Sharon's voice began to return fully to normal. Following the wedding, improvement tended to occur only during the latter part of the day. After about a week of this pattern and about a week of occasional 'croakiness', her voice problem vanished. She said this occurred at a time when, having taken the step into marriage, she was feeling more confident about her relationship with Kevin, of expressing her views and of showing her independence. In particular, she felt that she was able to be a woman in her own right and that Kevin had accepted and adapted well to this. Thus, she said, she was relieved to find her worst fears unfounded. Because of her new found confidence in herself, she had also been able to be more outspoken and to confront both her employer, who was making unreasonable work demands, and other staff members who had been treating her badly. As a consequence of speaking her mind in this situation, she was much happier at work and this stress greatly diminished. There had been a significant decline in her depressive/anxiety symptoms and, shortly after, she was discharged from treatment.

Summary

This chapter has described factors commonly found in psychogenic voice disorder and has illustrated the type of strategies that can be used in treatment. Factors often associated with psychogenic voice disorder are high levels of anxiety, acute or chronic life stresses, interpersonal relationship or marital difficulties, personal overcommitment or assuming the onus of family responsibilities, difficulties in setting appropriate personal and interpersonal limits, inhibition concerning the expression of thoughts or feelings and associated high levels of helplessness or powerlessness.

In considering these factors, we described how in a cognitive–behavioural treatment approach the therapist would select an appropriate combination of strategies from the following possibilities: anxiety or stress-management training (providing information about autonomic arousal, training in basic relaxation skills, self-monitoring, 'thought catching' and evaluation of thoughts, positive self-instruction, diaphragmatic breathing and rapid relaxation); target setting; record keeping; guided evaluation or analysis of dysfunctional or negative thinking; guidance in challenging unhealthy thinking and finding healthy alternatives, sometimes employing cue cards which summarise positive thoughts; giving information about the nature of stressful life events; giving advice; marital therapy focused on improving communication and rewards in relationships; role playing and assertiveness training (expressing feelings, setting limits, resisting coercion from others); and behaviour modification techniques such as prescribing a half-hour worry period and programmes employing operant conditioning principles.

It was stressed that, when successful, the techniques described above can directly increase feelings of personal control and self-confidence and that positive changes in these areas have been related to reduced feelings of anxiety and depression. A selection of case examples were used to illustrate both the psychological factors associated with psychogenic voice disorder and the therapeutic strategies employed.

Chapter 6
The Application of Cognitive–Behaviour Therapy in Speech and Language Therapy

As we have highlighted a number of times throughout this book, there are many areas of the speech pathologist's work where it is necessary for the therapist to be concerned with the patient's psychological adjustment and to consider a psychological dimension within the treatment. This is particularly true where it is recognised that a degree of cognitive and/or behavioural change is required for the patient or patient carer in order to support a healthy therapeutic outcome. In the introduction to their text *Helping People Change* Kanfer and Goldstein (1982) stress that a good treatment programme requires clearly conceived treatment goals and that we can differentiate between the following five treatment objectives which are not mutually exclusive:

> (1) Change of a particular problem behaviour, such as poor interpersonal skills; (2) insight or a clear rational and emotional understanding of one's problems; (3) change in a person's subjective emotional comfort, including changes in anxiety or tension; (4) change in one's self-perceptions, including goals, self-confidence, and sense of adequacy; (5) change in the person's lifestyle or 'personality restructuring', an objective aimed at a sweeping change in the client's way of living.
>
> *(p.8)*

It can be appreciated that any of these five treatment objectives could be applicable to a wide range of patients managed by the speech pathologist, including the patient with a psychogenic voice disorder.

While the focus of this book has been mainly on relating the use of cognitive–behaviour therapy to the treatment of psychogenic voice disorders, the same model of treatment may be usefully applied to many other fields in which the speech pathologist works. Once the speech pathologist is familiar with the methods of assessment and treatment which were explained in Chapters 4 and 5, the basic principles of the therapeutic method can be applied to a wider range of communication disorders and to new situations. In this respect, this final chapter will further illustrate, through case examples, the application of the therapeutic method to psychogenic voice disorders and will consider a wider range of communication disorders in which speech pathologists will have the opportunity to apply cognitive–behavioural treatment strategies. For the latter we have chosen stutterers, trans-sexuals and hearing-impaired individuals to provide examples of patients whose problems are very different from those of patients with psychogenic voice disorders, but where cognitive–behavioural techniques can be used. In addition, we will describe how cognitive–behaviour therapy may be useful in dealing with common problems experienced by the carers of neurologically impaired patients. Finally, we provide a brief critical overview highlighting some of the limitations inherent in the cognitive–behavioural approach.

Table 6.1 provides a list of cognitive and behavioural strategies that we have applied both in the work with treating psychogenic voice disorders and to a range of speech and language disorders.

Table 6.1 Cognitive and behavioural techniques useful in speech and language therapy

Stress management training	Relaxation training
	Rapid relaxation
	Self-monitoring
	Training in diaphragmatic breathing
	Record keeping/target setting
	Positive self-instruction
Specific cognitive strategies	Training in observation of negative thoughts
	Challenging negative thoughts
	Looking for alternatives
	Selecting and practising positive self-instruction
Assertiveness training	Role playing and rehearsal
	Expressing feelings and emotions
	Graded practice and task assignment
Highlighting the ABCs	Patient education or demystification
	Therapist/patient collaboration in planning for change

The examples in this chapter of the communication disorders to which this model can be applied, together with the suggested treatment strategies, are not exhaustive. Our intention is simply that these examples should encourage the speech pathologist to view cognitive–behaviour therapy as a potential tool for effecting change with every individual and at any stage of a patient's management.

Psychogenic voice disorders

In working with both dysphonic and aphonic patients, when a direct symptom-modification approach provided by voice therapy does not reap results, cognitive–behaviour therapy has proved to be a promising therapeutic method. If the common psychosocial characteristics of people with a psychogenic voice disorder (which were discussed in Chapter 1) are perpetuating the voice disorder, then these underlying features and behaviours in the patient need to be addressed primarily. The advantage of the speech pathologist being skilled in cognitive–behaviour therapy has been discussed in the Preface, whilst the speech pathologist's expertise in voice therapy ensures that, while working at a psychological level, the therapist does not lose sight of how the voice is functioning. The voice can be observed by the speech pathologist and advice given, and there may be a time during the cognitive–behaviour therapy when it is appropriate to intervene with direct voice therapy. It may, for example, be the case that once cognitive and behavioural changes have taken place which may alleviate the precipitating causes of the voice disorder, then direct voice therapy will be necessary to re-educate the voice from its habitual misuse to normal functioning. Nevertheless, as suggested in the Preface, in the initial work the speech pathologist is advised not only to seek further training but also to seek a degree of clinical supervision from a psychologist who is familiar with the cognitive–behavioural method.

Although we have some reservation about attempting to use cognitive–behaviour therapy with conversion voice disorders, it was seen in Chapter 1 that true conversion disorders are rare. Therefore, this therapeutic method has application for many aphonic patients.

The value of the psychological interview was seen in Chapter 4. The speech pathologist's ability to know what questions to ask, how to ask and what to listen for is vital for eliciting the essential information and then for formulating a treatment plan. When working with a patient with a voice disorder, the speech pathologist may find that significant information is disclosed after several sessions of treatment. It is important to be alert to this and to vary the treatment strategies accordingly. The ability to recognise what information is significant, knowing when to probe for more information and what treatment strategies are appropriate is not something which comes easily or automatically. However, once the therapist is fully conversant with the cognitive–behavioural interviewing and treatment model – to the extent that these consciously shape the way the therapist is construing the cause and possible treatment of problems – then, with time and practice, it becomes easier not only to distinguish 'the wood from the trees' but to develop effective treatment programmes.

The following four cases provide examples of cognitive–behaviour therapy applied to patients with voice disorders. In these and the case studies that follow the speech pathologist may recognise familiar strategies – particularly the more behavioural techniques. However, prior to selection of the treatment strategies, the cognitive–behavioural model has allowed the speech pathologist to assess more of the causative factors through recognising the contribution that thoughts have to emotion and behaviour. This, then, provides a more complete view of the various factors maintaining the patient's problem and encourages the speech pathologist to draw on multitreatment strategies. Thus, while it may appear on the surface that many of the treatment strategies are really quite simple, they could not have been chosen without first acquiring a more comprehensive picture of the patient's problem.

Case study: Gladys

Gladys was a 65-year-old lady referred to the speech pathologist from the ear, nose and throat department; she had no obvious laryngeal pathology, except that adduction of the vocal cords was not complete on phonation. Her voice had been initially aphonic for seven weeks, although she had a history of intermittent loss of voice since the age of 18 years.

During the voice assessment Gladys acknowledged that the periods of aphonia were associated with times of stress. The recent aphonic episode coincided with her return from a holiday in Australia, where she had been visiting her daughter. On assessment, she was observed using a strained dysphonic voice characterised by harsh, breathy quality with raised pitch and occasional phonation breaks. She complained of excessive tension and aching in the larynx. She described several other symptoms of tension, notably bad sleep patterns and occasional migraine, but mostly reported being 'a worrier', saying: 'I worry over other people, not myself'. This theme of caring for others was pursued by the speech pathologist's questioning and it emerged that Gladys had been the eldest of eight children and that she had largely brought up her younger brothers and sisters. Gladys had left home when she was 17 and she said that her mother, who died two years previously, never forgave her for leaving. This caring role had been perpetuated for Gladys and she mentioned various family members and friends who looked to her for support. In particular, she was living at home with her husband and 44-year-old son, both of whom relied on her. Her husband had had a stroke 13 years previously and since that time his moods had been unpredictable. Gladys felt that she couldn't blame him for his bad temper and that she had got used to avoiding confrontation and to 'bottling things up'. Her son had not worked since an accident seven years previously and would not move out of the house until his compensation claim had been settled. Her one close friend, in whom she had been able to confide, had died 5 years previously.

From this assessment there was enough information to suggest that Gladys was used to shouldering the responsibility for many family members and the stress of this was reflected in the timing of her recent aphonia, which began the day she returned from a carefree holiday. She was not used to expressing her own needs and there was some conflict over speaking out, in that she elected to bottle things up rather than challenge her husband's difficult behaviour. The speech pathologist tentatively pointed out the coincidence of the recent voice loss with the return home and Gladys was willing and able to gain some insight into the relationship between home stresses and her voice disorder.

The speech pathologist planned six sessions of therapy to include direct voice therapy, thorough relaxation training, breath control and voice work for an expanded vocal tract, together with teaching some assertiveness skills and encouragement for Gladys to recognise her personal needs and to find a balance between meeting these needs and taking responsibility for others. Gladys was seen over a seven-week period.

It was in the first therapy session that Gladys complained of a severely aching throat and she identified that tensions with her son that morning had caused her voice to deteriorate and feel constricted. She thought that it was her relationship with her son that was her main stress and this became a prime focus in therapy. She was encouraged to discuss the difficulties, which amounted to the fact that she would like him to leave home but she felt that she couldn't ask him to do this because she feared that he would react stubbornly and 'go off and sleep rough'. As his mother, Galdys felt that she had to do the best for him and she couldn't risk him neglecting himself if she asked him to leave home; however, this caused a tension for her because, in reality, she would have liked space for herself and her husband. The speech pathologist encouraged her to voice her feelings more to her son and suggested that it was not unreasonable to enquire about his plans for finding a place of his own. The speech pathologist talked to Gladys about the need for a balance of 'give and take' in a relationship and suggested that, if she were looking after her son too well, he had little motivation to behave differently. She was asked to think of ways of broaching with her son the subject of his future plans and also to begin to set some limits on what she did for him and some expectations of what he would do for her. The session ended with a brief introduction to relaxation training.

Following the first session, Gladys had her first full night's sleep for years and the work on relaxation training was repeated and extended in the next two sessions. Gladys was quite quickly making both cognitive and behavioural changes at home. She had talked with her husband about the relationship between stress and her dysphonia. As a consequence he had been supportive and had had a quiet word with her son to explain this to him. Thereafter, her son had been more amenable, although their communication remained limited. Alongside this, Gladys began to try out more assertive behaviour as opportunities arose. The speech pathologist gave her permission to value herself and to find a balance between fulfilling her own needs and caring for her son and husband. Instead of staying in at home until after lunch, Gladys told her son what there was to eat and he prepared it himself. When an opportunity came for her and her husband to have a weekend away, she took it willingly and had no misgivings about leaving her son. She returned in good spirits and with normal voice for the first time, pleased also that her son had been responsible for himself.

Because her son did not volunteer conversation, Gladys would fall in with him and this sometimes left her feeling depressed and frustrated. An example of this was that to get to the hospital for her appointments in speech pathology she had a rather complicated journey by bus; alternatively her son could drive her. They began to get into a pattern of Gladys worrying about the journey and not knowing whether her son would offer to drive her, then at the last minute he would say that he would or would not do so. As a result she arrived once or twice feeling angry that he had played this game with her. This behaviour was discussed as symptomatic of the poor communication between them and of Gladys's reluctance to express her needs or to risk offending her son. It was suggested that the following week Gladys should take the initiative to ask her son whether or not he would be able to drive her, so that then she could make her own plans. If he declined, then she could at least prepare for getting the bus and would be saved the worry of uncertainty about her travel arrangements. This strategy worked well and she began to find that, as a result of her being more assertive, her son was more cooperative and they were able to plan the travel arrangements. She found that, if her son began an argument, she could walk out of the room as if she wanted no part in it and, generally, she found the atmosphere in the house easier.

As far as their communication went, Gladys described her son as a loner and as someone who spoke little to people. He had few friends, but he enjoyed photography and animals. She had been surprised when he showed an interest in some photographs she had taken of wild animals. In order to build on their relationship the speech pathologist suggested that she could try opening conversations with him that were related to his interests in animals and photography.

One further target set by the speech pathologist was for Gladys to write a list of things that she might like to do for herself. The example was given that this might be a small desire, such as window shopping in the town, but the suggestion was to encourage Gladys to think of herself. Although Gladys showed some resistance to this task, indicating that she didn't feel it needed to be done, she returned the following week with a list and was surprised to find that it had been a useful exercise. This was the sixth session, by which time Gladys had made obvious cognitive and behavioural changes. She felt more in control of her relationship with her son and she found that they were able to live more comfortably together. She said that she had been doing things that she wanted to do, for instance decorating a room, and said 'I'm not worried about anyone else, not so much anyway'. She said that she had really been given the chance to think differently about things and that she felt a changed person.

Her voice had been normal for three weeks but she was aware that it would croak if she became stressed. However, here too she felt confident and commented that, if her voice did deteriorate, she would be able to ask herself what was causing it.

Case study: Mary

Mary, a 70-year-old widow, was referred to the speech pathologist from the ear, nose and throat department with aphonia. She gave a history of intermittent dysphonia and aphonia since the previous Christmas, 10 months earlier. In the July following she was assessed by the otolaryngologist and, subsequently, was admitted to hospital for stripping of her thickened left vocal cord. She was then instructed to have five weeks voice rest, after which time her voice was very weak and dysphonic. By the time that she was referred to the speech pathologist, in October, her voice was virtually aphonic with some tense, high-pitched phonation and she complained of pain and aching in her throat.

From assessment it was clearly evident that she had many stresses in her life and that these were largely related to two of her three sons. One son had become bankrupt before the previous Christmas and she had felt personal humiliation and worry, in part because she was a shareholder in the company. She was concerned not only for her other son, who was alcoholic, but also because his wife was abusive and badly behaved towards her. Mary had been widowed for 15 years and lived alone. She had not talked with other people about either of her sons because she found it too painful. Mary admitted that she was a worrier and tended to bottle up anxieties. This was because she did not like to be seen to be complaining, in case other people found her tiresome. Therefore she would put on a brave face and would worry on the inside. She seemed to have a tendency to put others before herself and this was explored in a later session when she explained that, when she was a newly married young woman, she and her husband had lived with her mother-in-law, who was very domineering. Consequently, Mary said she had grown accustomed to being 'trodden all over'.

In recent months Mary had been feeling tearful and depressed and this had added to her loneliness, since her symptoms caused her to avoid company. However, she remained quite active with some senior-citizen groups. Unfortunately, in these situations she was finding her aphonia stressful since it made talking difficult. She reported that in the past when she had been run down or worried she had experienced brief periods of voice loss.

Initially the speech pathologist attempted to regain phonation through a variety of vocal tricks and techniques. Although phonation was heard on a spontaneous cough and laugh, the speech pathologist was unable to facilitate primitive phonation; indeed, the attempts resulted in Mary hyperventilating. Direct voice work was therefore put aside and for the first three sessions the speech pathologist taught relaxation, encouraged discussion of her main worries and suggested the technique of evaluating her 'good and bad' worries (see Chapter 5). When Mary discussed her worries, these were actually more immediate stresses that had arisen in her social network, rather than being related to her two sons. The main worry that Mary expressed was related to a friend. They would talk every day on the telephone and it emerged that this person was controlling Mary and her behaviour suggested that she was jealous when Mary went out without consulting her. Since Mary didn't like to upset her friend she tended to appease her. It appeared that this situation was frustrating and depressing Mary and two therapy sessions were spent discussing the relationship. In the first, the speech pathologist explained the importance of having a balanced relationship, where Mary felt equally important and able to voice her own feelings. At the same time, since her friend seemed to feel threatened and jealous of Mary, the speech pathologist suggested that Mary reassure her friend that she valued her friendship and that going out and seeing other people did not detract from this. Mary was also asked to list her worries in order that she could start to identify what was depressing her and so that she could work together with the speech pathologist to find coping strategies. The discussion regarding her friend resulted in Mary trying out some assertive behaviour during the following week. When her friend began complaining to Mary, she firmly told her how she felt. Mary also decided to telephone her when she wanted to, not when she thought she ought to. She said that she no longer felt compelled to apologise all the time to her friend nor did she feel guilty about seeing other friends. She reported that her assertive behaviour resulted in her friend becoming more respectful of her. This encouraged Mary to try out assertive behaviour with other people. Primarily, this involved telling the person how she felt or expressing her view.

Between sessions Mary had identified and written down her good and bad worries and the speech pathologist then focused on how she might tackle her worries. Good worries were described as worries where positive steps could be taken to change things. One example of a worry which Mary had identified was the need for her to go to the dentist. On discussion it was clear that Mary had a fear of dentists –

dating back to bad experiences as a child. She also felt rather embarrassed that the dentist would see she had let her teeth get into such a bad state of decay. At the same time she was worried that she might lose some teeth if she did nothing. These conflicts provided the opportunity to discuss 'negative cognitions' and to identify negative self-talk. The speech pathologist suggested that, since Mary's fear arose from her experience with the dentist as a child, she could expect practices to have changed radically since that time; in particular pain relief was now much superior. The speech pathologist also reassured Mary that dentists would be accustomed to looking at bad teeth and her case would be no different. Furthermore, it was explained that going to the dentist did not commit Mary to having any dental treatment and she could accept or refuse this as she liked. Exploring this particular worry provided an example of how Mary might examine and challenge her negative thoughts, consider positive self-statements and look for practical steps to dissolve her worries. Thus, she was asked to examine the other worries on her list in a similar way.

In subsequent sessions, Mary reported positively on how she was finding solutions to her good worries. There was also further opportunity for the speech pathologist to discuss these and, in particular, to demonstrate changing negative thoughts to positive ones. In this process a theme which became increasingly apparent was that Mary had lost confidence in herself. Although the assertive behaviour was giving good results, she continued to have a number of self-doubts. One example, which came up in a session, was that she had bought a new coat but would not wear it until all her family had approved it. She felt sure that they would criticise it. This gave the speech pathologist the opportunity once again to explore with Mary how negative beliefs and thoughts, for example, 'I know my family won't like this coat', can be unhealthy and how she could change these to positive statements, such as 'I like this coat; there's nothing to suggest my family won't like it too, but, even if they don't, it doesn't matter because I do'.

During these first three sessions Mary's voice varied and often during discussion it would become much more normal. Although therapy was not focused on the voice, as Mary reported success in her assignments and as her relationship with her friend improved, it was pointed out that her voice too was improving. As is sometimes the case with patients with psychogenic voice disorders, as with other stress-related disorders, a major life stress did not emerge until the fourth session. In all probability it was this stress that had triggered the dysphonia and the other stresses were contributory.

In the fourth session Mary was able to explain further why she thought she had lost her self-confidence and why she was always apologising. She spoke for the first time about her third son and explained that four years ago his wife had 'taken against her' and treated her badly. They had not spoken for three years, until last Christmas, and during that time Mary had had almost no contact with her son and grandchild. (In this session Mary was initially aphonic, but as she spoke openly of this feud her voice returned.) Over the past year Mary's daughter-in-law had changed towards her and now seemed to be wanting to restore their relationship. However, Mary could not fully trust her and, in particular, still harboured hurt and angry feelings about the earlier treatment. Nevertheless, anxious not to offend and set their new relationship back, she swallowed her feelings and was going out of her way to comply with the wishes of her daughter-in-law, even when it did not really suit her. (Note how, inadvertently, her compliant behaviour through fear of offending had created additional feelings of resentment.)

Initially, the speech pathologist responded by reflecting that Mary's daughter-in-law had behaved unreasonably in the past and that Mary appeared to have good reason for feeling hurt and angry. (Many patients need to hear that it is perfectly acceptable to have negative feelings and that they should not feel guilty about this. Ideally, however, they need to find better ways of dealing with the feelings than trying to suppress them.) However, while the reasons for her daughter-in-law's behaviour were not clear, it did seem that she was trying to rebuild a relationship with Mary. Here again, the speech pathologist suggested that, when working at their best, normal relationships need to be balanced and that Mary and her daughter-in-law had to find that balance without Mary becoming controlled. Because Mary had had success in being assertive with other people, and because her assertiveness had not caused those relationships to deteriorate, she felt almost ready to put this into practice with her daughter-in-law. Following a rehearsal in the session concerning what to say and how best to say it, she was able to set limits with her daughter-in-law and express some of her hurt feelings during the following week. At the next session, a week later, her voice was virtually normal. The session reviewed positive self-statements, expressing feelings and setting limits with other people. At this point Mary was planning a three-week Christmas holiday with her son and daughter-in-law and was feeling hopeful and confident about her developing relationship with her daughter-in-law.

Although this treatment example is not yet completed, it seems to illustrate how cognitive and behavioural changes can take place in a short, six-week, period, and that in this case, as these changes took place, so the voice improved.

Case study: Louise

Louise was a 19-year-old student referred to the speech pathologist by the ear, nose and throat department with small bilateral vocal nodules. She had a history of recurring tonsilitis and infections of the upper respiratory tract and had been placed on the waiting list for tonsillectomy.

During the assessment session it became clear that both her singing and speaking voice had 'fallen off' over a period of two years, but there had been a more rapid deterioration over the previous eight months. Louise's voice was hoarse and deep with phonation breaks and she complained of tenderness and aching around the larynx and a sensation of 'pins and needles'.

Louise's parents were both involved in music professionally and she had been singing since the age of six. She was now in the second term of her first year of a music degree and living away from home. She had chosen singing as her first subject and piano and flute as her second and third options. She showed pleasure in talking about her course and openly acknowledged that singing and music were very important to her. Her ambition she said was to become a professional session musician.

Louise's lifestyle was hectic and demanding and voice use was excessive and unrealistic in terms of work and social commitments. Her personality was outgoing and she had a non-conformist, 'punk' style of dress. The course demanded a lot of her time because she had chosen a particularly ambitious combination of options, including practical workshops, study and lessons. Louise was at the same time a lead singer in a folk band and had undertaken voluntary extras, e.g. musicals and shows at college. She commented 'There is something happening every month.' Socially, Louise spent a lot of time in smokey, noisy atmospheres, particularly pubs and house parties. In addition, prior to the sudden deterioration in her voice, she had been regularly busking with friends. Based on all this information she agreed that she did seem to be 'burning the candle at both ends'.

Louise was very worried about her music course and her future and tension was evident in her posture and jaw. A course of six weekly sessions was agreed, after which progress would be reviewed and discussed. The interval between appointments in fact varied considerably because of interruptions.

Louise was given an explanation of and information about the formation of vocal nodules and its connection with vocal misuse and abuse and with her particular lifestyle. The therapeutic style was initially largely symptom-based to reduce and eliminate her unhealthy vocal habits, to encourage more awareness of a healthy relaxed vocal tract and encourage more awareness of caring for and monitoring a healthy voice. Therapy included relaxation training, breath control and voice exercises; Louise was already being taught the Alexander Technique at college for postural problems.

During the first two sessions, her voice began to improve. The concept of 'overuse' of the voice and physical and mental exhaustion in all aspects of her life were discussed.

A three-week break in therapy arose at this point because of the planned tonsillectomy. Contact with the singing teacher at the music college supported the speech pathologist's impression of a student who was non-conformist externally and very talented, but who was pushing herself to her limits and was highly anxious and worried about her voice.

Following removal of her tonsils, Louise was feeling low about her voice and her speaking voice had deteriorated slightly in quality from the previous session. With further questioning she was able to confirm that her singing was beginning to improve, but her speaking voice was very tight with laryngeal and jaw tension. The focus of the session was on relaxation training, both general and specific, and on breath and voice exercises to encourage a more relaxed vocal tract.

After a further three-week break in therapy due to non-attendance, Louise returned to clinic with a deep, hoarse voice with phonation breaks. She had been out socially the night before and had drunk heavily and overused her voice shouting and in company with her friends. She was still feeling down about her voice and its apparent deterioration and was extremely anxious. It was at this point that the speech pathologist decided to alter the emphasis of therapy from a more symptom-based approach to a more psychological approach. Sufficient information had been amassed with regard to the causative factors which could be described using the three *P*s (see Chapter 4) as follows:

Predisposing factors

- Strongly held belief about acceptable 'rough' speaking voice and lifestyle factors.
- No awareness of difference between relaxed and tense voice.
- Desire to be a successful singer.

Precipitating factors

- Increasingly excessive voice use related to lifestyle.
- Beginning a music course.

Perpetuating factors

- The music course led to: fear of failure in singing exams, the apparent conflict of a desire for a 'smooth' singing voice with a 'rough' speaking voice, increased vocal demands.
- Increase in tension resulting in habitual voice strain, constricted vocal tract and insomnia.
- Negative thoughts about first, failing exams, second, her voice quality and, third, being unable to realise her ambition as a vocalist.
- Maintaining her initial core belief that a rough speaking voice is preferable.

In order to increase her insight into her problem and allow her to adopt a more rational approach to solving her voice disorder, Louise was asked to keep a daily diary for one week to include detailed voice use in any situations involving worry or stress. She was not asked to grade her voice because she was already over-anxious about voice quality. (The speech pathologist who works with the professional voice user will recognise the care needed in dealing with this group because much is vested in the voice and consequently there is much to lose if it becomes faulty.)

Louise was also asked to write a list of worries and to try to identify which were productive worries, i.e. those where a solution could be found with some thought, and unproductive worries where no solution could be found no matter how much worry (see Chapter 5).

It was agreed that therapy would only be effective if some continuity could be achieved and subsequent appointments were arranged at weekly intervals. Voice quality at the following and next two appointments was significantly improved and Louise was more relaxed in posture and around the jaw and larynx. She commented that she had enjoyed meeting the targets from each session and that it all made sense to her. The daily diary confirmed the exhausting lifestyle and this visual record helped her to recognise for the first time the extent of her unrealistic expectations for herself, both at college and socially. With this increased awareness she was able to acknowledge the need for changes to break the pattern of vocal abuse and her motivation in therapy increased.

Louise's list of worries was primarily related to her voice disorder and about changes in accommodation. The latter was being dealt with and she was therefore able to see an end to this worry, but she was unable to address the worries about her voice and this in turn created increasing stress and tension. One worry was that she would not be able to take her practical singing exam at the end of term. This had led on to further negative thoughts such as 'My voice is terrible. I'm never going to sing properly again. I'm going to fail the course and music is the only thing I'm interested in.'. Possible solutions were discussed as to how to end the exam worry. Discussion with the speech pathologist allayed fears about approaching the tutor and risking further bad news, i.e. that she would still have to sit the exam. The situation was only hypothetical and it was agreed that it was better to know the truth and to deal with that. Louise decided to speak to her tutor and the speech pathologist would also make contact if this was felt to be necessary thereafter.

The daily diary and list of worries further highlighted a number of conflicts. Louise's voice was very important to her and yet she continued a lifestyle that perpetuated the voice disorder. This conflict led on to a discussion about her self-perception and how she viewed herself.

She described herself as outgoing, loud and impulsive, but at the same time sensitive, routine and meditative. She enjoyed both noisy modern music and classical and 'serene' music. She wanted a clear, pure-tone singing voice, but liked the slightly rough speaking voice and cultivated a local accent because it had 'character'. She was happy with her relationship with her parents and described them as 'alternative', but 'very prim' and 'well spoken'; she didn't want to sound like this. Further exploration of her relationship with her parents was not carried out because progress was being made.

The speech pathologist suggested that Louise listen to friends that she admired and whom she considered outgoing personalities, decide what it was she liked about their voices and their speech and note any differences. At a later date, she was set a target to discuss voice variations with her friends in order to seek their views with regard to acceptable voice quality.

Louise was also asked to use self-monitoring of her thoughts and to begin disrupting worrying thoughts about her voice by questioning their validity and by using rapid relaxation and deep breathing. At subsequent appointments she was able to comment that she realised that speaking-voice quality was not as important to personalities whom she admired as she had thought and that other non-verbal characteristics were equally as important. In discussion with her friends about voice qualities, she was surprised to find that they did not share her stereotyped views, rather that they appreciated that a wide variation in voices was acceptable. Also significant was that she had altered her perception slightly about personalities whom she admired and that, to her surprise, not all had the same vocal characteristics. She was able to clarify that 'loudness' of voice was still important to her but not as important as before.

Louise had resolved her worry about the singing exam by talking to her tutor and it had been agreed that she would not have to take the exam and that she would pass on earlier performances that academic year. This ending of worry had helped reduce tension. Further targets were set and it was agreed that she would cut out drinking binges completely, as well as late nights, and that it was all right to talk with normal volume and occasional loudness without strain.

Following one further session with continued focus on beliefs about personal lifestyle and what would be acceptable alterations in speaking voice quality, therapy was halted for exams. The relaxation programme was emphasised as important throughout this period and some rehearsal of positive self-statements about voice improvement were advised.

After a three week break, Louise attended for an appointment. Her singing voice was improving considerably in range and flexibility and she was feeling more confident about the possibility of full recovery of voice.

An ear, nose and throat examination four months post-referral confirmed that the vocal nodules had almost disappeared, with only slight changes at the junction of the anterior third and posterior two thirds of the vocal folds. Further indirect laryngoscopy four months later confirmed a normal larynx.

At a review appointment following this, Louise was relaxed and positive about her voice and more aware of setting limits for herself vocally and generally. Her speaking voice quality was still mildly hoarse with a slightly low pitch, but with no laryngeal discomfort or tiring. She had been able to accept some changes in lifestyle with some cognitive restructuring, but without compromising her personality. She explained that at the start of therapy she had not been able to understand the concept of a relaxed voice, but now she had an awareness of the contrast between relaxed and tense voice. She could now accept that a relaxed voice need not conflict with her self-image and that people's voices vary. In that respect her thinking was less stereotyped and she was less judgemental of others. She was less influenced by peer pressure and more sure of herself and what she wanted for herself.

In effecting these changes, the speech pathologist had found that the cognitive and behavioural strategies had been helpful; in particular the cognitive and behaviour targets, the daily diary and challenging and replacing the disrupting negative thoughts that she had had with regard to her dysphonia.

Case study: William

William, who was 67 and who worked in the entertainment world as a compere in clubs and as host on local radio programmes, was referred for a psychological assessment of a three-year dysphonia that had not responded to traditional treatment. His problem began when he was eating a steak and kidney pie and bit into a large piece of metal which cut his mouth and damaged his teeth. He also reported that the piece of metal started to go down his throat, that he could feel it 'turning' and 'getting lodged', and that he gagged and had to cough to bring it up. He felt that his throat had been scratched and his voice problem began following this incident. Extensive physical investigations at his local hospital and two London teaching hospitals failed to reveal any physical cause of his voice loss. Despite an extended course of voice therapy over many months and learning anxiety management skills, he never felt he made 'any concrete progress'. When seen for a psychological assessment, William was continuing to use the breathing and voice exercises taught during voice therapy but reported that, although this helped for a short while, the improvement faded rapidly. At the time of assessment he presented as a voluble, anxious, mildly obsessional man. His voice sounded harsh and strained and had little volume. Daily ratings of voice quality showed a typical pattern of poor quality for most of the day but with two or three half-hour periods of improvement. He noted that this improvement was usually associated with being relaxed and in a conversation which absorbed or interested him. He estimated that there was a more than 50% chance of the voice improving at these times. He noted that difficulties in raising his voice often caused anxiety and this usually made his voice deteriorate further.

At the first interview a psychological assessment was made of the thoughts which passed through his mind when his mouth was cut by the metal object and when he felt that his throat had been scratched. Although this had occurred three years ago, he could recollect his thoughts quite clearly. During the moments of trying to clear his throat he felt panic and fear for his life. He recalled feeling shocked and wondering what he had done. His first thought after regurgitating the piece of metal was that his throat had been scratched and then he thought about what would have happened if he had swallowed the sharp metal fragment. Emotionally, he reported feeling extremely distressed. Shortly after the incident, a number of people commented on his lucky escape and a companion wondered aloud about what might have happened if he had given the pie to his young grandson, who occasionally joined them at lunch. The thought of this provoked further anxiety and emotional distress. The assessment suggested that these thoughts added psychologically, as well as emotionally, to the physical trauma which he had experienced to his mouth and throat.

In the event of a life-threatening physical and emotional trauma of the sort William had experienced, we would expect an instinctive, self-protective, muscular constriction around the throat. A response of this type can easily become habitual since memories surrounding the incident, a heightened sense of personal vulnerability and further anxieties about being physically damaged while eating or having a similar incident happen again will stimulate the instinctive constriction. This view was supported by the fact that since biting the metal object, William had become very conscious of what he ate and swallowed. For a long period after the incident, he ate only mashed and finely chopped food and three years later could only eat meat if it was sliced into extremely small pieces. When William was asked to keep a daily record of his meals and to rate the difficulty he had in eating different types of food, it showed that he was never relaxed or happy when eating and that there was nothing he could eat without it causing him at least some difficulty.

This case illustrates the importance of a more broadly based, cognitive–behavioural, approach to treatment rather than focusing just on voice therapy. The psychological assessment suggested that it was extremely likely that a major factor maintaining the muscular constriction in his throat was the daily effort he was making in trying to eat. The phobic anxiety around swallowing would be provoked on each occasion of eating, causing the constriction reflex to be reinforced and strengthened with time. As a result of this element in the maintenance of the voice disorder, it would be appropriate to develop a desensitisation programme that aimed at reducing the anxiety surrounding eating and swallowing. Once this was tackled and the anxiety and conditioned muscular reflex reduced, he would be more likely to benefit from voice therapy and breathing exercises. Thus, for William, the initial focus of treatment was progressive muscular relaxation, training in rapid stress control techniques, and a graded *in vivo* programme of maintaining a relaxed state while eating and swallowing. William cooperated well with the programme and, over time, felt the approach did make eating and swallowing easier with some foods. However, in this particular case, even after lengthy treatment, many meals remained difficult for him to eat and his voice problem was unaltered. It was felt that there were a number of ongoing external stresses which at the time inhibited progress (for example, a court case and anxieties about receiving compensation for his loss of employment etc. since the incident), as well as other significant factors which made treatment difficult. The latter will be described later in this chapter when the reasons why some patients fail to benefit from cognitive–behaviour therapy are considered.

The stutterer

We have already described Fransella's (1972) finding that stutterers have difficulty construing what it means 'to speak fluently' and how they can also have difficulty identifying themselves with being fluent. Her findings suggest that treatment should be directed primarily, or at least initially, toward changing personal constructs, cognitions or self-concepts surrounding being and not being a stutterer. However, this cognitive focus should be part of a broader integrated therapeutic programme. Thus, irrespective of the cause of the stutter, or when self-concepts about being or not being a stutterer have already been or are now the focus of treatment, speech pathologists often gear their treatment of the dysfluent patient to helping the person gain control over speaking situations. This is advocated in differing approaches by, for example, Van Riper (1973), Perkins (1973) and Ryan and Van Kirk (1978).

Typically a stutterer will build up fear and avoidance of certain situations and will anticipate failure in effective communication or a worsening of the dysfluency. For example, the stutterer will anticipate blocking on the telephone because he or she has done so in the past. Cognitively, the stutterer may assume that the listener will be judgemental and the consequence of blocking may be that the person feels humiliated and a failure. This can lead to fearful anticipation of making a telephone call, a range of stress-induced physiological changes (e.g. racing heart, sweating, increased breathing rate, shallow breathing, tensing of laryngeal musculature, general body tensing), emotional changes (high level of anxiety associated with telephone use) and avoidance behaviour. Past experience of failure and expectation of failure can also foster learned helplessness (Adams, 1983) and this expectation may even be generalised to the therapy situation.

In addition to the above factors, we also find that some stutterers have difficulty forming relationships and cannot view their relationships in equal terms. In these cases, the person usually undervalues him/herself and has a low self-image or anxieties surrounding self-presentation. Typically, people who are important in the stutterer's life – those construed by the stutterer to hold positions of authority, for example, parent, teacher, boss – create the most difficulty for the stutterer when he or she attempts to form equal relationships.

With these issues in mind, cognitive–behaviour therapy may be of use with stutterers and can be applied in either individual or group therapy. Within Van Riper's therapy, for example, the cognitive–behavioural desensitisation programme aims to reduce the patient's negative feelings about stuttering. Van Riper recognises the value of assertiveness training in achieving this end, as well as the effect that this has on counteracting anxiety in the stutterer. We have also found that using cognitive–behavioural assertiveness training, in order to enable stutterers to act more confidently in both speaking and non-speaking situations and to help them reconstrue their position in terms of equality, is a great benefit to many people who stutter.

Treatment example

Objective

The objective of the treatment is to improve the patient's self-confidence, self-esteem and assertiveness, particularly when talking on the telephone, and therefore to reduce the anxiety experienced in this situation and help the patient gain self-control when speaking.

Assessing the problem

When assessing the patient, the speech pathologist may consider the three Ps, described in Chapter 4, in relation to the patient's behaviour and thoughts in speaking situations. We could hypothesise that the assessment of a difficult speaking situation, such as talking on the telephone might look as follows:

Predisposing factors:

- Dysfluent speech that becomes worse when the patient is anxious.
- Poor self-image and difficulty in valuing self on equal terms with others (probably reinforced by dysfluency).
- Previous failure when speaking on the telephone.

Precipitating factors:

- Cognitive and behavioural reactions, for example, a strongly held belief that the attempted telephone call will result in failure; belief that the listener will be judgemental; and the increased autonomic arousal.

Perpetuating factors:

- Predisposing and precipitating factors lead to poor task performance, which reinforces or confirms feelings of failure and inferiority.

This assessment of the patient's thoughts and behaviours would be arrived at using observation, questioning and record forms, as described in Chapter 4. The speech pathologist would simultaneously assess the speech characteristics using his or her preferred assessment tools and methods. In this way, the speech pathologist builds up a comprehensive picture of the stutter and the stutterer. In particular, attention is paid to events that exacerbate the stutter and to the thoughts, feelings and behaviour of the stutterer before, during and after these events. Whilst developmental and past experiences will be valuable information to collect, as we emphasised in earlier chapters, the focus will be on finding out more about recent circumstances and current difficulties.

Applying the technique

1. Initially, the speech pathologist needs to help the patient understand the problem more fully and to evolve an agreed or shared view of the difficulty. This is necessary preparation for the patient to accept the rationale of the treatment intervention. The patient will be presenting his or her own view of the problem and it is up to the speech pathologist to listen to that view and to define the problem in terms that are acceptable to both of them. The speech pathologist's explanation to the patient that the difficult speaking situation has resulted from a learned behaviour may help to demystify the problem for the patient and may encourage him or her to believe that a changed response is possible.
2. At a behavioural level the speech pathologist would introduce relaxation techniques and would instruct the patient in the use of these,

first in the absence of a telephone, second when imagining or rehearsing making a telephone call, and finally when practising a telephone call. This would be graded in difficulty in order to gradually desensitise the patient to the situation and to help him or her in the effort to gain control. The cue reminders, for example the 'red dot reminder', described in Chapter 5, would be useful strategies for helping to establish general and rapid relaxation training. It should be noted here, however, that there is a school of thought that finds relaxation training of limited value for stutterers; patients either do not find that relaxation is of any value when they are blocking or their anxiety levels are too high to be able to employ relaxation techniques. Heide and Borkovec (1983) state that in 5% of patients relaxation leads to an increase in anxiety. These findings highlight how important it is to consider individual differences when developing a treatment programme and why it is usually necessary to employ more than one treatment strategy.

3. As therapy gets under way, the speech pathologist will begin to help the patient identify his or her own irrational and negative thoughts before, during and after making a telephone call. The intention is to guide the patient in challenging these thoughts and replacing them with more rational or more constructive thoughts. The speech pathologist encourages the person to ask 'What am I telling myself that is upsetting me?' Having identified the automatic thoughts, the patient is asked to examine them for cognitive distortions (exaggerations, generalisations etc.) and to offer a more rational and constructive response. For example, since the patient is likely to have been focusing on the worst possible outcome, the speech pathologist can encourage him or her to question how likely or accurate this fantasy really is and to list alternative outcomes. The speech pathologist may encourage the patient to observe his or her thoughts and to use the sort of self-questioning suggested by Aaron Beck (see Chapter 5, p.83). It can be useful to ask the patient to write down his or her automatic thoughts during the therapeutic session in order for these to be explored, further understood and questioned. The speech pathologist can then encourage the patient in the use of positive self-instruction which we also described in Chapter 5 (p.82). In this way, the patient may learn to replace an automatic cognitive response with a more realistic interpretation of the situation.

In Table 6.2 we offer an example of the patient's negative thoughts prior, during and following a telephone conversation, together with the patient's revised positive thoughts. The speech pathologist would usually help the patient explore the negative thoughts and put the more realistic and rational responses to the test through role play or

Table 6.2 Stutterer using telephone: recording and challenging negative automatic thoughts

Negative thoughts	Positive thoughts
Before	
I can't make this telephone call because I will stutter and the listener will think I'm stupid	I may stutter, but if I do it doesn't mean that the person will automatically think I'm stupid nor that I am stupid
I know I'm going to make a fool of myself on the 'phone so there's no point trying	There's a chance I will stutter, but I will do my best and nobody's perfect
Each time I talk on the 'phone it makes me feel inferior	Why associate having a stutter with inferiority? It's a nuisance. It sometimes makes communication more difficult, but it doesn't make me inferior. I shouldn't make a silly value judgement
During	
He thinks I'm stupid	He may not think I'm stupid. Even if he does that's only his viewpoint. I know that I'm intelligent
He's interrupting and making me feel stupid	He's probably interrupting because he thinks that's helping me. I need to keep calm and continue the conversation to the best of my ability
I feel so tense and anxious. I'm going to die	Of course I'm not going to die. Relax, I'm going to do my best and I know I'll feel good about that afterwards
After	
That was a disaster. I feel really embarrassed	That was difficult, but I got through it. I don't feel embarrassed because I have every right to talk even if I'm not always fluent
I know he thinks less of me now	I don't know he thinks any less of me. After all, he's only human and he's probably got 'failings' of his own

rehearsal. The patient could role-play a pretend telephone conversation with the speech pathologist and, after each attempt, discuss how successful he or she had been in practising the positive self-statements and the effect this had on his or her emotions. The speech pathologist would also discuss with the patient the effects at a behavioural level, for example body tension, stomach butterflies and fluency of speech.

Once rehearsed and prepared, assignments can be planned for real-life practice between appointments. Flexibility and creativity are neces-

Date	Anxiety	Negative thoughts	Positive thoughts	Fluency
2.7.92	70% anxious sweaty, butterflies.	I'm going to make a fool of myself.	That's an assumption. I don't know I'll make a fool of myself. I'll just do the best I can and see what happens.	Blocked twice, otherwise managed to say what I wanted.

Figure 6.1 Form for recording the results of practice assignments when using the telephone

sary for the therapy programme to be individualised and the speech pathologist should help the patient draw up an individually tailored record sheet like the example shown in Figure 6.1.

Case study: Rosemary

Rosemary was referred to a speech pathologist because of a mild stutter. She was 42 years of age, worked as a health visitor, and was separated from her husband. She had two children and for the past six years she had lived with her daughter, who was then 17.

Rosemary's stutter began when she was five and a half years old. Her family travelled widely and her first language had been Spanish before she learned French at the age of three. This was to be her main language until the age of ten, when she switched to English. When her stutter began she recalled that she was looked after by a Swiss nanny who used to hit her with a carpet beater and whom she described as 'strange'.

Despite a long period of treatment with a speech pathologist, extending over almost four years, and therapy involving a variety of approaches including desensitisation and block modification, personal construct therapy and deep relaxation with hypnotic suggestion, Rosemary's stutter did not improve. When desensitisation and block modification could not be progressed further, it was considered that this was because Rosemary was not sufficiently desensitised to her stuttering and not at a point where she could constructively handle confrontation of her abnormal speech. During the personal construct therapy a similar picture emerged, in which discussions concerning the physical aspect of stuttering were threatening and not therapeutically productive. What was apparent from observations and her own reports, however, was that the stutter was usually present when Rosemary was in the presence of someone who was authoritative and/or verbally intimidating or aggressive. These situations caused her considerable distress. Further therapy, including relaxation and hypnotic suggestion, only resulted in temporary improvement and setbacks. At this point, the speech pathologist referred Rosemary for a psychological assessment and, thereafter, she was seen in joint therapy.

The initial psychological assessment highlighted that, in addition to stuttering in situations where she felt intimidated, Rosemary stuttered most commonly when with her own family, her sister, her mother and her daughter. She felt there were two explanations for her stutter when with her mother and sister. First, she felt that her stutter had become habitual because she 'had always stuttered with them'. Second, she felt that she tried to say too much too quickly. Her other comments, that her sister and mother treated her as 'the baby' in the family, suggested that their attitude may also reduce her self-confidence and bring on her stutter. Analysis of Rosemary's stutter in the presence of her daughter suggested that it was largely caused by the tensions in their relationship. Thus, her stutter in this situation seemed to be mostly related to her difficulty coping with aggression or intimidation.

The initial step in treatment was to ask Rosemary to keep a record of situations where she began to stutter and to note occasions when she was in conflict with her daughter. At the next meeting her daily diary showed that the stutter occurred when she felt pressure to hurry through what she had to say and that at these times she became tense and had most difficulty when placing the emphasis or stress on a harsh syllable. The diary also showed that the stutter was worse when two or three people were talking to her at the same time and when she had to organise people, give orders or be directive. The one area of conflict with her daughter was particularly related to difficulty with assertiveness. Rosemary was mainly concerned with the fact that her daughter was unhelpful around the house and she had not found a way of changing this behaviour.

At this session Rosemary was given guidance in using positive self-instruction to resist the impulse to hurry through what she had to say, and it was suggested that she use this when dealing with conflicting demands on her attention as well as when being assertive. She was also instructed in diaphragmatic breathing and rapid relaxation to reduce her tendency to become tense at these times. The session also explored her difficulty with her daughter and how the latter might be confronted over her lack of input into running the household. Rosemary agreed to speak to her daughter if she was unhelpful and to consider making a contract in which her allowance was given on condition of help around the home.

At the following meeting Rosemary reported beginning to implement the above suggestions. She had told her daughter that she intended to restrict her allowance unless she did more around the home and her daughter's response had been to be more helpful. Rosemary had not introduced a formal programme to reinforce her daughter's helpful behaviour, but she reported that she had given a lot of thought to how this would be done if it was necessary and her comments suggested that she had a good grasp of how to carry it out appropriately. However, assessment at this session indicated that she had not really communicated to her daughter how pleased she felt about her improved behaviour. The therapist therefore focused on how to give more feedback and praise to her daughter. At a review session six weeks later Rosemary reported that she had been able to follow the advice of giving feedback and praise. The relationship with her daughter was much improved and her daughter had continued to be more helpful.

At this session Rosemary wanted to talk about her concern over having to give two talks to her colleagues at work. She was worried that she would have breathing difficulties and would stutter or dry up completely. The psychologist suggested that she prepare her talks and spend time alone regularly rehearsing the presentation in her imagination. In doing this, she was instructed to create positive images of herself coping with anticipatory anxiety prior to the talk, as well as using positive self-talk related to speaking slowly and keeping relaxed, diaphragmatic breathing, self-hypnotic techniques and rapid relaxation during the presentation. She was also instructed to practise presenting her talk out loud when she was on her own at home, in order to help her get used to projecting her voice and to have some real-life practice at monitoring her speed of presentation and using positive self-instruction. At the end of the session Rosemary said she was anxious about not having gained enough from the hypnotic procedure to ensure success in this endeavour. It was therefore agreed that over the next few weeks she should apply the procedure outlined above and, if she then continued to feel that she needed more help in becoming fully relaxed, she would then be taught progressive muscular relaxation.

Because of a missed appointment, Rosemary was not seen until after she had given her talks. However, it did not appear that the appointment had been necessary, since she reported benefiting considerably from the rehearsal and, consequently, the presentation had gone very well. Since, however, these experiences had nonetheless been rather stressful and since she felt that she tended to be tense in general, Rosemary still felt that she would like further training in stress management techniques. She was therefore provided with a pre-recorded audio tape of progressive muscular relaxation instructions and seen three weeks later in order to take her systematically through the steps involved in rapid stress control (i.e. self-monitoring, positive self-instruction, diaphragmatic breathing and rapid relaxation).

Rosemary was seen again at a four-month follow-up and reported that the anxiety management techniques had been very helpful. She had applied them successfully in a number of stressful situations and she felt they gave her much more control over her tendency to stutter. She did not feel the need for further psychological help with her stutter.

The speech pathologist felt that Rosemary had more self-knowledge and could face up to her stutter more readily; consequently, she felt that she had at last arrived at a point where she might be able to respond to more conventional stuttering therapy. Indeed, Rosemary was enthusiastic to work on fluency techniques. At this time Rosemary moved from the area and the speech pathologist transferred her case and recommended a course of therapy based on Van Riper block modification.

The trans-sexual

Speech pathologists who become involved in the management of the male-to-female trans-sexual will be familiar with the tendency that these patients have of feeling dissatisfied with the level of success they have achieved in presenting as a woman. The trans-sexual's frequent complaint is that her voice is predominantly responsible for preventing her from being perceived by others as feminine. Typically, the patient will look to the speech pathologist for reassurance that she is convincing. In such an instance the patient needs to become more reliant on her own self-appraisal and to be less self-critical and negative in her assumptions, in other words, to be more realistic and positive in her thinking.

Treatment example

Objective

The objective is to build the patient's confidence in her success in the feminine role and to make it possible for her to use her feminine voice successfully and to communicate unselfconsciously.

Assessing the problem

Initially the speech pathologist will have undertaken a thorough assessment of the patient's communication and will have instigated an appropriate course of treatment in order to maximise the patient's success as a female speaker. To date, treatment advice with regard to voice therapy for the trans-sexual is not extensive and we refer the reader to Greene and Mathieson (1989) and Chaloner (1991). The speech pathologist's objective is not confined to raising the pitch of the voice, but extends to helping the trans-sexual present as a feminine speaker. Therefore, apart from modifying features of the voice and speech, the speech pathologist is concerned with non-verbal features and with social skills.

The speech pathologist explores with the patient the degree of confidence that she has when speaking and any reasonable and unreasonable dissatisfaction with her success. Again, the three Ps, employed earlier with the stutterer and discussed in Chapter 4, provide a useful framework for assessing what the trans-sexual feels about her self-image, her effectiveness as a female speaker and what is going wrong in speaking situations.

Applying the technique

1. The speech pathologist explains that what we tell ourselves in situations, and our interpretation of other people's responses, affect how we feel about our performance. To illustrate this, the patient is encouraged to discuss the feelings and thoughts that she experiences before, during and after a speaking encounter. This should reveal any irrational and negative thoughts. The speech pathologist will need to discover whether the patient has more difficulty communicating comfortably with certain people (for example, men) or in certain situations. Beginning a daily diary will usually provide helpful information, particularly when the patient is uncertain about which situations are most worrying.
2. Through graded role play with the speech pathologist and later in real-life situations, the patient can practise conversations and the use of positive self-instruction. Table 6.3 illustrates the change in cognitions which the patient might achieve through the discussion and rehearsal.
3. The trans-sexual also needs to become reliant on self-appraisal rather than remain dependent on the speech pathologist's rating of her success. Thus, in addition to the cognitive strategies described above, the speech pathologist may encourage the patient to rate her general level of success in a speaking situation. The speech pathologist might create a record chart (see Figure 6.2) that would link the specific treatment for voice and communication with the patient's evaluation of her level of performance in a speaking situation. Alternatively, an assignment could be set up – as shown in Figure 6.3 – where the patient scores her overall success, as well as thoughts and feelings related to a specific speaking situation.

Through this careful observation of both her speech and her thinking, the patient should become more realistic in her self-appraisal. Altering

Table 6.3 Trans-sexual in speaking situations. Recording and challenging negative automatic thoughts

Negative thoughts	Positive thoughts
Before	
I'm no good as a woman. It's obvious to everyone that I'm not really feminine	I've got so far with my female identity and a lot of people believe in me. I shouldn't assume that I know what other people are thinking
My voice is going to let me down	My voice is a bit deep, but I know a lot of women have deep voices and they still pass as feminine
During	I'm doing my best as a woman and even
She thinks I'm a fraud and that I'm really a man	if I'm not perfect it doesn't follow that other people think I'm odd
Everyone's staring at me, they're about to find out I'm not a real woman	It's natural for people to look at you when you talk. If I can think about the conversation and listen to their response, I'll relax and enjoy the conversation rather than feel so self-conscious
After	The person I was talking to gave me no
I wasn't any good as a woman	reason to think he noticed that I was a transsexual. This probably means I'm quite convincing as a woman
I felt so self-conscious it was dreadful	I was a bit self-conscious but I still enjoyed talking to that person. We seemed to get on well and he appeared to take me for a woman. So it wasn't 'dreadful' and I don't really need to feel self-conscious

```
Speech/Communication              Date/Event              Rating
                                  16.2.92.
                                  Talking to shop assistant
Voice, pitch                                              6/10
Voice, modulation                                         -
Voice, quality (soft, breathy)                            5/10
Apparent eye contact                                      8/10
Relaxed posture                                           6/10
Overall success                                           6/10
```

Figure 6.2 Self-rating of speaking situations: 1 = very little success; 10 = complete success

Date/Event	Rating /10	Thoughts and feelings
18.2.92.	7/10	Had a good conversation with stranger in the hospital. We got on well and I really liked talking to her. I felt that she completely accepted me as a woman. My voice was a bit deep, but it didn't seem to matter.

Figure 6.3 Recording success in speaking situation

negative thinking to positive thinking can help her be more satisfied with her level of success in communication, despite limited change to her vocal features. In this way the patient may become less preoccupied with her male-sounding voice and more confident in her overall success as a female speaker. The cognitive, emotional and behavioural changes each reinforce the others. If the patient feels more hopeful and confident about the speaking situation, she is likely to feel less anxious, her communication will probably be more successful and this success can lead to more positive, more realistic assumptions about future social encounters.

Case study: Stephanie

Stephanie was a 45-year-old male-to-female trans-sexual. She was referred to the speech pathologist prior to her reassignment surgery. She worked as a lecturer in a College of Further Education and she was to continue in the same job after her transition to the female role. Stephanie had a course of voice therapy prior to the surgery and a subsequent course five months after the surgery.

Despite positive adjustments in her speech, throughout the voice therapy Stephanie expressed insecurity in the female role. She continued to feel that her voice betrayed her male side and she had a fear of being 'found out' to be a man. Her self-reflections were rather contradictory; on the one hand she spoke positively about her achievement of a feminine voice and on the other she asked for constant reassurance that she sounded feminine and for the speech pathologist to rate her voice. The speech pathologist recognised that, in addition to continuing direct work on the voice, it was necessary to explore how Stephanie really felt about her new voice and her new female role and to offer counselling that would enable Stephanie to become more self-reliant and accepting of her female speech and behaviour. Although Stephanie had made changes at a superficial behavioural level to her voice and speech, and she had developed some insight into her problems, she needed to change in her self-perceptions and in particular her self-confidence and sense of adequacy. Without this change Stephanie was likely to attribute any difficulty in speaking situations to failure in sounding convincing as a female. This would perpetuate a sense of dissatisfaction with her voice. The speech pathologist recognised that there was a danger of the direct voice therapy being sabotaged by Stephanie's inclination to lengthy discussion about her insecurities and feelings. If this was allowed to happen, then the teaching of new voice skills was likely to be jeopardised. Therefore an agreement was made between the speech pathologist and Stephanie that three sessions would be directed to refining aspects of female voice and communication and the fourth session would offer the opportunity to discuss how she was feeling about her voice and to plan further therapy, if it were necessary, in order to explore her adjustment to the female role. The three sessions of voice work were productive and gave Stephanie further confidence in her abilities. By this time she was presenting well in the female role and had achieved a lighter voice with more forward focus, which was perceived as higher in pitch. During these sessions the speech pathologist was alert to comments Stephanie made about her success in communicating outside the clinic. Repeatedly she would report great success in some speaking situations and devastating failure in others. The speech pathologist hypothesised that the success or failure of a speaking situation in Stephanie's opinion was influenced by what she was telling herself before and during the encounter. The fact that she had more success with some of her new students than with some of the old students and with her teacher colleagues suggested that she might have preconceived ideas and fears about how people who had known her as a man might be viewing her now, whereas one might assume that new students would not be suspecting or critical.

Towards the end of the third session Stephanie was invited to talk about how she felt in speaking situations and the speech pathologist reflected that what we tell ourselves, our 'self-talk', influences both our behaviour and how we feel inside. Stephanie confirmed that this might be happening, 'If I go into the situation with the right attitude, I do much better.'. The speech pathologist then recalled one of the comments that Stephanie had made in the previous session with regard to a conversation she had had at work, when she had said, 'I was devastated, it was a complete disaster.'. Stephanie was asked to recall that incident, who she had been talking to and why it was, in her opinion, such a disaster. She related the encounter which had taken place with a group of students at College. She explained that she had felt nervous in their company, that they could not accept her transition to the female role and she willingly agreed that she had expected the fear and humiliation that she felt. She was able to reflect that these were frequent emotions in encounters with certain groups of people, whereas 'at home, in a "clean slate" situation, I do well 99% of the time and at worst I'll get a polite tolerance and probably the benefit of any doubt'.

In the speech pathologist's opinion, improvement in the difficult speaking situations and in Stephanie's confidence as a female speaker depended on Stephanie's ability to be able to identify what it was that she was telling herself and to attempt to challenge irrational self-talk and replace it with rational responses. This was discussed with Stephanie and an observational record sheet was drawn up (Figure 6.4). Stephanie was asked to observe herself in three encounters over the following two weeks and to write down some of her 'self-talk' and some of her feelings on the record sheet.

Date and situation of encounter	Before	During	After

Figure 6.4 What am I telling myself and how do I feel?

When Stephanie returned she had recorded four situations and time was spent in discussing these. The speech pathologist was able to summarise that there seemed to be three themes that emerged from these recordings. First, Stephanie feared talking to men; for instance before one encounter she had written 'Hesitated twice. Will it be a man?' and during another encounter with a husband and wife she had written 'I know I could more confidently chat to the wife', and afterwards had written 'Big worries persist where men are concerned.'. Second, her performance was better when she believed in herself and especially in her appearance. She had referred to her appearance in several situations, for example before one she had written 'Ultra-confident re. appearance' and that conversation had been a success. During another situation, which was potentially confrontational – she was complaining to a store manager – she found that her appearance influenced her ability to be assertive and she wrote, 'I know that my appearance was very good and other people (in the store) believed in me, so why shouldn't he?'. On a third encounter she had recorded failure and had written afterwards 'I wasn't happy with my appearance beforehand – I lost control completely'. The third feature of these recordings was that Stephanie still believed that her voice let her down and she had made comments during and after some of the situations with regard to the control she felt she had over her voice.

The speech pathologist explained to Stephanie how self-talk affects behaviour and perceptions. In her case she needed an opportunity not only to identify what she was telling herself, but also to challenge irrational thoughts and replace these with more rational and positive responses and she needed an opportunity to practice more assertive behaviour. Stephanie accepted the offer of four further sessions of therapy, which would develop this area. The speech pathologist then prepared a treatment programme which Stephanie was given. In this way the objectives were explicit. For example, one main objective written in the programme was:

> Encourage positive self-statements and self-rating when talking. To practice real speaking encounters and to modify any self-criticism with positive self-talk. To learn to rate yourself favourably.

At this time Stephanie had come to the conclusion that her position at work was becoming impossible and she began to consider leaving the College where she taught. Once this had been voiced by Stephanie, the speech pathologist was able to reflect that it had been an ambitious decision to remain in the same employment and that a change in environment could be positive, since it would allow Stephanie a fresh start.

In the following month Stephanie made her decision to leave and, subsequently, began to look for alternative employment. This resolution, once she was no longer struggling to win respect at work from people who had known her as a man, helped Stephanie to be more settled.

Prior to the first appointment to implement the new treatment programme, Stephanie enthusiastically recorded 56 speaking situations! This provided the groundwork for the first appointment, which was spent reviewing her successes and failures. Of these 56 encounters Stephanie recorded only eight as failures and these were with men and with teenage girls. Stephanie reported that she found it impossible to talk with teenage girls because they were so suspecting. With prompting Stephanie did recognise that some of the successful encounters had included teenage girls; indeed the 48 successful encounters had included a wide range of people, male and female, from all walks of life. She demonstrated that she was already becoming more assertive and self-confident with men. She said that there had been a couple of very bad situations with men, but added: 'I was quite pleased with the way I handled those. I certainly wouldn't have done it three to four months ago; I would have taken flight'. Instead, she stood her ground and told herself 'It's his problem; everyone else here is happy with me'. Thus, even though Stephanie had not yet practised positive self-statements in the clinic, the previous discussions about the need to replace negative self-statements with more realistic, positive statements was influencing her behaviour.

The speech pathologist then prepared Stephanie for a practice assignment that would involve talking to the hospital receptionist. In preparing for this, Stephanie acknowledged that her self-talk was negative: 'Oh my God, how old is she going to be – will there be people watching?'. She needed some prompting to find a more realistic message to replace this, but chose: 'I just have to do my best, regardless of her age. Just because she may be young doesn't mean to say it won't go well.'. After the assignment Stephanie recounted her thoughts as follows:

Before: My first thought was that she was younger than I remembered.

After: My voice wasn't as light as it could have been. She wasn't as convinced as she could have been, but I might be wrong there!

The speech pathologist pointed out the tendency that Stephanie had to give herself negative messages. The homework from this session was designed to help Stephanie move on to the next step. She was asked to record her self-statements before and during speaking encounters and to then change any negative statements to positive ones. Examples were suggested to her to demonstrate this.

During the subsequent two appointments, Stephanie demonstrated not only that she could construct more positive self-statements, but also that she could put them into practice. She recorded more speaking situations and some of these are noted in Figure 6.5. She was also given an opportunity to practice further assignments in the clinic.

By the end of the third session Stephanie was beginning to demonstrate a shift in her thinking. By recording her encounters and through challenging negative self-statements, she was becoming more confident and realistic. She was less fearful of young females and was not blaming her voice for everything that went wrong. She realised that the voice was not the only significant feature that implied femininity and indeed she was more realistic about how much she could expect of the voice; 'If I can't change the voice, I can concentrate on my manner and everything else.'. She became aware that when a situation began badly it need not finish badly and that she could regain her poise and confidence.

Stephanie continued to practise and explore speaking situations into the fourth session. By this time she was behaving with more self-confidence and was taking more responsibility for herself. There were times when she realised that either the voice or her social interaction was not 100%, but she was quick to balance any self-blame with a more rational viewpoint. Overall, she was by now more comfortable in the feminine role and was more convinced of her own ability and less concerned that other people would judge her poorly.

Situation	Before	During	After
Store purchase	They are <u>all</u> young in this section but I can and must present positively (i.e. positive manner/timing)	I'm winning because I'm being mindful! This is an OK one because I am confident. The voice is lowish and relatively poor now – I'm worried about others nearby.	Overall, my confidence and my effort were good. I kept talking to her even when I didn't have to, that worked. I lost a little in confidence in the middle but I need not have! Others around me were not too interested. Good!
Making an appointment with a new hairdresser.	I can't judge this one, I can't see what's going on inside the shop – but the day is going well and it need not change.	Oh God, it's more crowded than I thought; they are all young; it's quiet; they are all taking an interest... I've started this badly; I've avoided eye contact with the rest of them and 'wished them away'. I'm speaking too quietly and the quality has suffered. I have to stick with it and show her a confident manner and a smile or two, if I'm to recover this one – but I think I can.	It wasn't as good a performance as I would have liked but I didn't let my confidence drain away. I didn't minimise on the encounter to get it over with, I responded to her. It wasn't the best effort but I'm pretty sure it was still successful. Anyway, I can take away any margin of doubt I may have left when I meet her next because: 1. I can only do better. 2. I know what to expect.

Figure 6.5 What are you telling yourself?

In this case, the direct voice therapy had been necessary to equip Stephanie with the ability to alter her voice, but this alone had not been sufficient. The cognitive–behavioural strategies employed, in conjunction with the voice therapy, had enabled Stephanie to dig deeper and to gain insight into her thoughts and behaviour. It also gave her a better awareness of her abilities, which led to a shift in her self-perceptions, greater self-confidence and more assertive behaviour.

The hearing impaired

The following case provides a further example of how the speech pathologist can apply cognitive–behavioural principles to another client group.

Case study: Keith

Keith was a 63-year-old man with a ten-year history of Ménière's disease. He had a severe hearing loss and was helped to a degree by a hearing aid. He had retired from his job as a sales manager in a department store and he ran the home while his wife worked. He referred himself to the speech pathologist as he was anxious to maintain good speech. He seemed to lack confidence as a communicator and said that his speech deteriorated when he was talking to strangers. Although he did not avoid talking to strangers, for example shopkeepers, he disliked such conversations through fear of misinterpreting their speech. He reported difficulties controlling his loudness when nervous and also occasional instances when he momentarily 'lost his voice'. He was quite a proud man and did not like people to know that he was deaf.

Following a voice and speech assessment, the speech pathologist spent a session explaining voice and speech production and gave feedback to the patient about his own abilities. Keith was reassured that most aspects of voice and speech remained normal and three sessions of therapy were then agreed in order to allow Keith to monitor his loudness levels better.

In the first session Keith quickly got a grasp of quiet, normal conversational and loud voice and, over the week, he practised monitoring himself using these three levels.

In the second session the speech pathologist explained that they would now go out together into the hospital to practise conversing with people, so that Keith could monitor his loudness levels. He became anxious at the thought of this and so the speech pathologist role-played two or three examples with him first. He was able to rehearse what he was going to say, for example:

'Can you tell me the time please?'
'Can you tell me how to get to the hearing aid department?'

Together the speech pathologist and Keith went into the outpatient building and the speech pathologist directed Keith in the task. He was asked to approach a stranger, to ask a question and afterwards to discuss with the speech pathologist the appropriateness of his levels of voice. The first assignment went reasonably well, although Keith noted that, though he didn't hear the reply, he had pretended to understand without asking for a repetition. The speech pathologist encouraged him to ask for a repetition in future. The second assignment went well. On the third assignment in the hospital shop, Keith asked one of the two shopkeepers for the correct time:

Keith:	[to first woman] Could you tell me the time?
First woman:	It'll cost you!
Second woman:	[Keith not looking in her direction] Eleven fifteen.
Keith:	[anxious and agitated] Now I asked you [first woman] the time and you [second woman] answered.
First woman:	It's eleven fifteen.
Keith:	[without hearing the time] Thank you very much.

When discussing the assignment Keith was clearly angry. He said that it was exactly the kind of situation that he had to deal with, that the women were rude and he didn't understand the response.

The speech pathologist and Keith returned to the clinic and discussed his reaction. The speech pathologist acknowledged that it might not have gone to plan, but it was a real-life situation. She encouraged Keith to reflect on his response and how he had felt. He verbalised his thoughts, 'She was rude and she made me feel angry and stupid.'. The speech pathologist explored with Keith why he had not asked for a repetition or disclosed his deafness. It emerged in the discussion that he had high expectations and standards for himself and considered it a failure to admit to any disability. He felt that other people would judge him negatively and think less of him if they recognised that he was deaf. This acknowledgement triggered two memories that he had of bad encounters where he was mimicked for being deaf. The speech pathologist suggested that other people's bad behaviour need not have a lasting or damaging effect on Keith. For example, if the woman in the hospital shop was really rude, then he might reflect that 'she was rude, but that's her problem.'. The speech pathologist pointed out that what was important was for Keith to come away from speaking encounters feeling good about himself and feeling that he had done his best. The speech pathologist also pointed out that, rather than believing that the disclosure of deafness betrayed a failure in himself, there could be advantages in alerting people to his deafness so that they are given the opportunity to respond more sensitively.

Following this discussion the speech pathologist suggested that they review the encounter in the hospital shop and they then explored alternative responses which he might have tried. The speech pathologist took the lead by suggesting various possibilities:

1. 'I'm sorry, I didn't hear you, I'm deaf.'
   Keith disliked this response; he said that it reinforced his feelings of inadequacy and that having to say sorry made him feel submissive.

2. 'I can't hear you, can you say that again.'

This second response also made him feel uncomfortable because it evoked a guilty feeling for placing the blame on the speaker.

3. 'Would you mind saying that again, I didn't catch it, my hearing's not very good.'

   Keith was pleased with the last suggestion. He thought it was both assertive and courteous and said that he would feel comfortable trying it out.

The speech pathologist also advised Keith on the importance of keeping calm and of speaking more slowly with strangers.

At the end of this session the speech pathologist instructed Keith to record five speaking encounters over the next month and to aim for more assertive responses.

When Keith returned a month later there was a very definite change in his behaviour. He was more self-confident and very positive about speaking situations. First, he had decided to carry around a card with the three points previously discussed.

1. Keep calm and relaxed.
2. Speak slowly.
3. Tell people if you haven't heard.

Although he read this from time to time, having the instructions in his pocket seemed to act as an *aide memoire* and gave him a feeling of security. He then recounted the five assignments that he had attempted and reported that they had all been successful. He had initiated four of the speaking encounters. On one occasion, when he had not heard the response, he deliberately remained calm and gave himself time to think of the speech in context so that he could guess the words he hadn't heard. He had been so pleased with the ease with which he was conversing that he set up a potentially difficult situation with a shopkeeper who he knew was quietly spoken.

The confidence which Keith had gained was evident and he said that he no longer felt irritated by other people's responses; indeed, he now looked forward to talking with people rather than dreading it. Keith happily acknowledged this change to a more assertive and confident behaviour and said he believed it would be a permanent feature in him.

Having reinforced the behavioural and cognitive techniques and having congratulated Keith on his obvious success, the speech pathologist arranged a further review appointment in six months. When Keith returned for the review he had maintained the changes. He recalled one example in a shop where he had become fleetingly aphonic. However, he had recognised this as tension at the time and, after composing himself outside the shop and talking to himself positively, he made a point of returning to buy something else. His voice was then normal and he was able to report a feeling of confidence at his perseverance and then success.

At this point Keith felt ready to discontinue therapy. In the speech pathologist's opinion, although Keith had initially sought advice to improve his speech intelligibility, what he needed was more an awareness of where he was going wrong with his communication and assertiveness skills in order for him to make better use of his good speech abilities.

The neurologically impaired

Helping the spouse, partner or carer

Professionals who take a holistic approach to managing a patient with acquired neurological impairment will be concerned with the reactions and role of the spouse, partner or carer. Some common difficulties that the carer may experience are: denial of the problem; having unrealistic expectations for their partner's recovery (their expectations being either too high or too low); changed feelings towards their partner (these may include strong feelings of dislike and resentment); feelings of helplessness and hopelessness; and adopting an over-protective role (thereby limiting their partner's independence and exposure to normal life situations).

In each of these scenarios there are ways in which cognitive–behavioural techniques can be applied.

Changing unrealistic expectations

Where there are unrealistic expectations on the part of the carer, the speech pathologist will need to focus on deepening the carer's insight and improving his or her understanding of the problem. To achieve this the speech pathologist will have to provide both clear explanations and concrete examples to which the carer can relate. Implicitly and explicitly, the speech pathologist will be outlining the parameters of expectation for improvement or non-improvement. If the prognosis for improvement is minimal, then the speech pathologist can present the prognosis in the most favourable terms. For example: 'Although tongue and lip movements are very poor, if you look at these assessment results they give an overall intelligibility rating of 50%. So, if you listen carefully, a conversation is possible. It may take a bit more concentration on your part, but as long as background noise is avoided and you look at each other when talking, you will be able to understand half of what is said'. In this way the carer is given a truthful explanation of the situation, encouraged to have realistic expectations and to think positively. By implication he or she is also being invited to help in the treatment regime. This can give the carer a positive role in his or her partner's adjustment and rehabilitation and may also reduce feelings of helplessness. Where possible the speech pathologist will want to share this information and understanding with the patient too. However, this may be difficult if the patient's cognitive dysfunction has reduced insight and understanding.

Changing negative feelings

Here it is important that assessment results are shared in order to empower the relative. Demystifying the disorder and providing a rational explanation of the patient's problems and behaviours is likely to be reassuring and may in itself change negative feelings.

In addition, however, ways should be found to encourage the carer to express his or her negative feelings about the situation. Most important in this is that the carer should be assured that 'negative feelings are very common and perfectly normal'. Once the carer realises that he or she is allowed to feel anger, resentment, dislike, etc. and has even been able to express these feelings openly without being contradicted or criticised by the speech pathologist, it is possible for any feelings of guilt to be eased. Success in this venture obviously requires at least basic training in counselling individuals who are in distress. In some cases a brief course of individual therapy may be necessary – particularly if negative cognitions are hard to shift – and introducing the carer to self-help groups or to other relatives may be recommended.

Changing feelings of helplessness and hopelessness

When the speech pathologist hears comments which suggest the presence of feelings associated with helplessness and hopelessness, the thoughts behind the feelings should be highlighted and explored with the aim of questioning what are usually false assumptions. For example:

Negative thought	*Rational response*
I can't cope.	Yes, it's awful but I have been coping so far. It's a huge adjustment but I've adjusted to life changes in the past etc.

The aim will be to instil a sense of not being helpless and a feeling that the situation is not hopeless.

Changing over-protective behaviour

Becoming over-protective towards the patient can lead the carer to be unnecessarily exhausted and indispensable. When the carer adopts an overly protective role the assumption is that he or she knows what is good for his or her partner and controls what the partner is exposed to.

Combining cognitive coping skills for the carer and implementing coping strategies for the patient at home may help the carer to loosen his or her control, to allow the patient more independence, whilst maintaining the carer's belief that he or she is still doing the best for the patient. For example:

Automatic, negative thought	*Rational, positive thought*
I can't go out any more because John is my responsibility and he can't function without me.	It's good for us to have time apart sometimes. The break will do me good and John will cope without me.
No-one else can look after John because they won't do it as well as me.	It's good for John to be with other people sometimes. If they do things differently to me, that doesn't have to be a bad thing. It may actually be good for John.

Implementing specific strategies for maximising speech or language ability would also help the carer cope. For example, simple aids for assisting recall problems might include:

- written lists, e.g. of things to do, people's names, shopping lists;
- dictaphone, e.g. patient or carer records the shopping list and patient replays this at the shop;
- carrying card with details to be remembered, e.g. a request for a bus ticket can then be read by patient or bus conductor;
- simple map for directions; this could be pictorial with easily identified landmarks;
- use of colour stickers; a sticker is put on certain objects around the house to provide a visual cue, e.g. toothbrush, medicine bottle, sugar jar.

These strategies will give the patient more independence and confidence and encourage the carer to feel less responsible for the patient's functioning. As the carer is able to withdraw from the over-protective role, the patient will be encouraged to be more self-supporting and adventurous. With growing autonomy the demands on the carer become less and so both mutually benefit.

A critical overview of cognitive–behaviour therapy

The intention in this chapter has been to convey how cognitive–behaviour therapy may be of potential value for speech pathologists in their many areas of clinical activity and we hope to have illustrated how it can be usefully adapted to new and various challenges. A relevant example of this in operation is that when the first author was initially asked whether psychological therapy could be offered for psychogenic voice disorder, he had no experience of working in this area. However, he assumed that the problem could easily be considered from a cognitive–behavioural assessment perspective and that, if this suggested specific patterns or causes (as described in Chapters 4 and 5), treatment could then be explored and evaluated. The results of these first collaborative steps in evaluation and treatment not only deepened and clarified our understanding of psychogenic voice disorder, but indicated that cognitive–behaviour therapy improves treatment outcome. Hence, we feel that it is possible that similar developments may occur in applying cognitive–behaviour therapy to other areas of speech pathology and these thoughts stimulated the writing of this chapter.

While we have selected and described specific problem areas for this chapter – psychogenic dysphonia, voice loss resulting from psychological trauma, stuttering, work with trans-sexuals, the hearing impaired and the carers of patients with neurological impairment – there may be other areas where cognitive–behaviour therapy can be applied. Having said this, we should caution that cognitive–behaviour therapy is not a panacea and it may be helpful to highlight briefly some of its limitations.

We have previously mentioned that simple counselling skills may be sufficient for a number of clients and that an understanding of cognitive–behaviour therapy may not be necessary for helping these patients psychologically. We have also mentioned that while cognitive–behaviour therapy can be a valuable approach when treating more complex problems, there can be factors which may mitigate against success. There are some situations when it is difficult to reduce stress (for example, the woman living with her dementing mother, whom we described in Chapter 5), and there will be occasions when, despite the most skilled therapeutic input, patients remain entrenched in their negative attitudes and behaviours.

There are also those disorders, like hysterical conversion and personality disorder, which do not readily respond to psychological therapy. The case of William, cited earlier in this chapter, may be another example of where, despite offering a deeper understanding of factors causing and maintaining the voice problem, cognitive–behaviour therapy may not alleviate the difficulty. In this case, assessment highlighted a number of post-trauma symptoms – recurring nightmares about the incident, long-standing general anxiety, irritability, distractibility, and a significant decline in sex drive – which, taken together, are typical of post-traumatic stress disorder. This condition, as its name implies, results from exposure to either a single traumatic or life-threatening incident or a number of stressful or psychologically disturbing life experiences. It occurs most commonly in survivors of major disasters, in war veterans and in those individuals, like William, who narrowly escape accidental death. Whilst psychological therapies can alleviate this condition, it can be extremely difficult to treat or resolve. Although phobic anxiety usually responds well to therapy involving relaxation and graded exposure, phobic reactions are more difficult to treat when the conditioned response (for example, William's reflexive throat constriction) is established in the context of a life-threatening experience and where the person feels that in again carrying out the same activity his or her life may be genuinely at risk. In these cases progress involves confronting the perceived danger, trusting that whatever went wrong is unlikely to happen again and overcoming or inhibiting the conditioned fear reaction. Few sufferers find this an easy task.

The above points illustrate that, even when the speech pathologist has some knowledge of cognitive–behaviour therapy, there will be patients who will still require a psychological opinion and there will also be individuals who will not benefit as much as might be desired from this form of psychological treatment. Concerning the last point, it should also be added that there may be some individuals who, for one reason or another, require more extensive psychotherapy than is typically offered in cognitive–behavioural treatment.

Although, taken together, these points highlight limitations which can exist in applying cognitive–behaviour therapy, experience and research suggest that the patient for whom it has little or no value is very much in the minority. For example, post-traumatic stress disorder is a rare condition, even within clinical psychology, and will be even more rarely encountered in a department of speech pathology. Similarly, it is usually the more psychologically disturbed patient who requires extensive therapeutic help and the studies of psychogenic voice disorder cited earlier (Aronson et al., 1966; Butcher et al., 1987; House and Andrews, 1987) suggest that these patients are also rare. Thus, while recognising its limitations, we continue to feel that cognitive–behaviour therapy can be an important, adaptable, therapeutic resource within the field of speech pathology, where it has relevance for the majority of patients whenever problems are psychosocial and cognitive–emotional in origin and where psychopathology is not extensive.

Summary and concluding remarks

The skill of any practising speech pathologist is to recognise what the patient's difficulty is, to listen to what the patient or carer is not telling you, as well as to what he or she is, and then to find a therapeutic route that will lead to a positive and healthy change. Often we find that what is apparently the salient feature that needs to be changed, for example the voice or the stutter or the speech intelligibility, is not the significant feature that needs to be changed at all. Instead, once the less apparent areas of behaviour or thoughts are changed, then either the more obvious symptom changes simultaneously or the patient's attitude to the problem changes. Such sequences of events have been demonstrated in each of the case histories, where we have seen that once the speech pathologist or psychologist has applied cognitive–behavioural techniques to a range of inner conflicts and external stresses, the presenting speech or voice disorder has either resolved or become less significant as a problem, or the patient has arrived at a point where it can be more easily treated by direct means.

In the Preface we recognised the importance of speech pathologists becoming equipped with counselling skills. The need for these skills within the field of voice therapy has been emphasised by Aronson (1990a, b) in particular. As described in Chapter 2, the training colleges in the UK stress that counselling skills are an essential ingredient in the development of every speech pathologist. Speech pathologists require these skills since, no matter what their sphere of work, they will be working to effect changes or adjustment to a problem.

We have presented cognitive–behaviour therapy as a model that speech pathologists might adopt in order to extend their counselling skills and become more sophisticated in their approach to psychological therapy. Cognitive–behaviour therapy has several advantages to speech pathologists over other methods. First, as was explained in Chapter 4, the approach incorporates Rogerian-style counselling skills and, currently, these are the psychological (or 'insight'-orientated) skills most frequently taught to speech pathologists. Second, speech pathologists are familiar with traditional behaviour therapy methodology and this part of the model can therefore be easily adopted. Third, the model is explicit and encourages patient collaboration, and it is structured, with targets set between sessions. All of this dovetails well with the speech pathologist's treatment plans and type of service delivery. As speech pathologists, we have found the model compatible with our knowledge base and by learning through collaborating in co-therapy with a psychologist we have become more familiar with the model and able to apply it in our work with other patients.

In this chapter we have described the various uses of cognitive–behaviour therapy in working with a wide variety of problems which present within speech pathology: psychogenic voice disorder, stuttering, voice work with trans-sexuals, treating the hearing impaired and helping the carers of patients with neurological damage. We have attempted to illustrate that, although it has limitations, cognitive–behaviour therapy has relevance in many cases. Whilst, in order that speech pathologists become proficient in the use of cognitive–behaviour therapy, we would advocate a learning period through either post-graduate training, co-therapy or supervision, we have aimed in this book not only to introduce cognitive–behaviour therapy as a working model within speech pathology, but also to encourage workers within the field to employ this method with patients with psychogenic voice disorder as well as with other speech and language disorders. We have found that the therapeutic rewards are considerable.

References

ADAMS, M. R. (1983). Learning from negative outcomes in stuttering therapy: 1. Getting off on the wrong foot. *Journal of Fluency Disorders*, 8, 147–153.

AMERICAN PSYCHIATRIC ASSOCIATION (1980). *Diagnostic and Statistical Manual of Mental Disorders*, 3rd edn. Washington DC: APA.

ARONSON, A. E. (1990a). *Clinical Voice Disorders*. New York: Brian C. Dekker.

ARONSON, A. E. (1990b). Importance of the psychosocial interview in the diagnosis and treatment of "functional" voice disorders. *Journal of Voice*, 4, 4, 287–289.

ARONSON, A. E., BROWN, J. R., LITIN, E. M. and PEARSON, J. S. (1968). Spastic dysphonia. I: Voice, neurologic and psychiatric aspects. *Journal of Speech and Hearing Disorders*, 33, 203–218.

ARONSON, A. E., PETERSON, H. W. and LITIN, E. M. (1966). Psychiatric symptomatology in functional dysphonia and aphonia. *Journal of Speech and Hearing Disorders*, 31, 115–127.

BANDURA, A. (1989). Perceived self-efficacy in the exercise of personal agency. *The Psychologist*, 2, 10, 411–424.

BARTON, R. T. (1960). The whispering syndrome of hysteric dysphonia. *Annals of Otology, Rhinology and Laryngology*, 69, 156–164.

BATES, G. W., CAMPBELL, I. M. and BURGESS, P. M. (1990). Assessment of articulated thoughts in social anxiety. Modification of the ATSS procedure. *British Journal of Clinical Psychology*, 29, 91–98.

BECK, A. T. (1976). *Cognitive Therapy and Emotional Disorders*. New York: International Universities Press.

BECK, A. T. and STEER, R. A. (1987). *Beck Depression Inventory*. Sidcup: The Psychological Corporation.

BECK, A. T. and STEER, R. A. (1990). *Beck Anxiety Inventory*. Sidcup: The Psychological Corporation.

BOONE, D. R. (1977). *The Voice and Voice Therapy*. Englewood Cliffs, N.J: Prentice-Hall.

BOONE, D. R. (1991). *Your Voice is Telling on You*. London: Whurr.

BOONE, D. R. and MACFARLANE, S. L. (1988). *The Voice and Voice Therapy*. Englewood Cliffs, NJ: Prentice-Hall.

BORKOVEC, T. D., WILKINSON, L., FOLENSBEE, R. and LERMAN, C. (1983). Stimulus control applications to the treatment of worry. *Behaviour Research and Therapy*, 2, 247–251.

BRADLEY, B. P. and THOMPSON, C. (1985). *Psychological Applications in Psychiatry*. Chichester: Wiley.

BRODNITZ, F. S. (1969). Functional aphonia. *Annals of Otolaryngology*, **78**, 1244–1253.

BROWN, G. W. and HARRIS, T. (1978). *Social Origins of Depression*. London: Tavistock Publications.

BRUMFITT, S. (1986). *Counselling*. Oxfordshire: Winslow Press.

BRUMFITT, S. and CLARKE, P. (1982). An application of psychotherapeutic techniques to the management of asphasia. In C. Code and D. J. Muller (eds) *Asphasia Therapy*. London: Arnold.

BURNS, D. D. (1980). *Feeling Good*. New York: Morrow.

BUTCHER, P. (1984). Existential-behaviour therapy: A possible paradigm? *British Journal of Medical Psychology*, **57**, 265–274.

BUTCHER, P. (1989). *Managing Anxiety: A Practical Guide*. London: Audio Arts.

BUTCHER, P. and ELIAS, A. (1983). Cognitive–behavioural therapy with dysphonic patients: An exploratory investigation. *The College of Speech Therapists Bulletin*, **377**, 1–3.

BUTCHER, P., ELIAS, A., RAVEN R., YEATMAN, J. and LITTLEJOHNS, D. (1987). Psychogenic voice disorder unresponsive to speech therapy: Psychological characteristics and cognitive–behaviour therapy. *British Journal of Disorders of Communication*, **22**, 81–92.

CARDING, P. N. and HORSLEY, I. A. (1992). An evaluation study of voice therapy in non-organic dysphonia. *European Journal of Disorders of Communication*, **27**, 2, 137–158.

CHALONER, J. (1991). The voice of the transsexual. In M. Fawcus (ed.) *Voice Disorders and Their Management*. London: Chapman and Hall.

COREY, G. (1991). *Theory and Practice of Counselling and Psychotherapy*. Monterey, CA: Brooks/Cole.

DARLEY, F. L. (1964). *Diagnosis and Appraisal of Communication Disorders*.Englewood Cliffs, NJ: Prentice-Hall.

DARLEY, F. L. and SPRIESTERSBACH, D. C. (1963). *Diagnostic Methods: Speech Pathology*. New York: Harper and Row.

DAVISON, G. C. and NEALE, J. M. (1978). *Abnormal Psychology: An Experimental Clinical Approach*. Chichester: Wiley. 2nd Edition.

DAVISON, G. C. and NEALE, J. M. (1982). *Abnormal Psychology: An Experimental Clinical Approach*. Chichester: Wiley. 3rd Edition.

DRYDEN, W. and ELLIS, A. (1988). Rational-emotive therapy. In K. S. Dobson (ed.) *Handbook of Cognitive–Behavioural Therapies*. London: Hutchinson.

DRYDEN, W. and GOLDEN, W. (1986). *Cognitive–Behavioural Approaches to Psychotherapy*. London: Harper and Row.

ELIAS, A., RAVEN, R., LITTLEJOHNS, D. and BUTCHER, P. (1989). Speech therapy for psychogenic voice disorder: A survey of current practice and training. *British Journal of Disorders of Communication*, **24**, 61–76.

FAWCUS, M. (1986). *Voice Disorders and Their Management*. London: Croom Helm.

FRANSELLA, F. (1970). Stuttering: Not a symptom but a way of life. *British Journal of Disorders of Communication*, **5**, 22–29.

FRANSELLA, F. (1972). *Personal Change and Reconstruction*. London: Academic Press.

FREEMAN, M. (1986). Psychogenic voice disorder: A multifactorial problem. In M. Fawcus (ed.) *Voice Disorders and Their Management*. London: Croom Helm.

FREEMAN, M. (1991). When is a voice disorder psychogenic? Some considerations for diagnosis and management. In M. Fawcus (ed.) *Voice Disorders and Their Management*. London: Croom Helm.

GOODKIN, R. (1969). Changes in word production, sentence production and relevance in an aphasic through verbal conditioning. *Behaviour Research and Therapy*, 6, 235–237.

GOSSOP, M. (1985). Drug and alcohol dependence. In B.P. Bradley and C. Thompson (eds) *Psychological Applications in Psychiatry*. Chichester: Wiley.

GRAVELL, R. and FRANCE, J. (1991). *Speech and Communication Problems in Psychiatry*. London: Chapman and Hall.

GREEN, R. (1990). *Survey of Counselling in Speech Therapy Special Interest Group*. Riverside Community Health, Bute Gardens Annex, London W6 7DR.

GREEN, R. (1992). Supervision as an essential part of practice. *Human Communication*, 1, 2, 21–22.

GREENE, M. C. L. (1972). *The Voice and its Disorders*. London: Pitman Medical.

GREENE, M. and MATHIESON, L. (1989). *The Voice and its Disorders*. London: Whurr. 5th Edition.

HARLOW, H. F. and ZIMMERMAN, R. R. (1959). Affectional responses in the infant monkey. *Science*, 130, 421–432.

HAWTON, K., SALKOVSKIS, P. M., KIRK, J. and CLARK, D. M. (1989). *Cognitive Behaviour Therapy for Psychiatric Problems: A Practical Guide*. Oxford: Oxford Medical Publications.

HAYHOW, R. (1987). Personal construct therapy for children who stutter and their families. In C. Levy (ed.) *Stuttering Therapies: Practical Approaches*. London: Croom Helm.

HAYWARD, A. and SIMMONS, R. (1982). Relaxation groups with dysphonic patients. *Bulletin of The College of Speech Therapists*, 359, 1–3.

HEIDE, F. J. and BORKOVEC, T. D. (1983). Relaxation-induced anxiety: Paradoxical anxiety enhancement due to relaxation training. *Journal of Consulting Psychology*, 51, 171–182.

HOLMES, T. H. and RAHE, R. H. (1967). The social readjustment rating scale. *Journal of Psychosomatic Research*, 11, 213–218.

HOUSE, A. O. and ANDREWS, H. B. (1987). The psychiatric and social characteristics of patients with functional dysphonia. *Journal of Psychosomatic Research*, 31, 4, 483–490.

HOUSE, A. O. and ANDREWS, H. B. (1988). Life events and difficulties preceding the onset of functional dysphonia. *Journal of Psychosomatic Research*, 32, 3, 311–319.

INCE, L.P. (1973). Behaviour modification with an aphasic man. *Rehabilitation Research Practical Reviews*, 4, 37–42.

INCE, L. P. (1976). *Behaviour Modification in Rehabilitative Medicine*. Springfield IL: Thomas.

JACOBSON, E. (1938). *Progressive Relaxation*. Chicago: University of Chicago Press.

JAREMKO, M. E. (1986). Cognitive–behaviour modification: The shaping of rule-governed behaviour. In W. Dryden and W. Golden (eds) *Cognitive–Behavioural Approaches to Psychotherapy*. London: Harper and Row.

KANFER, F.H. (1982). Self-management Methods. In F. H. Kanfer and A. P. Goldstein (eds) *Helping People Change*. Oxford: Pergamon.

KANFER, F. H. and GOLDSTEIN, A. P. (1982). *Helping People Change*. Oxford: Pergamon.

KAROLY, P. (1982). Operant methods. In F. H. Kanfer and A. P. Goldstein (eds) *Helping People Change*. New York: Pergamon.

KELLY, G. A. (1955). *The Psychology of Personal Constructs*. New York: Norton.

KOUFMAN, J. A. and BLALOCK, P. D. (1982). Classification and approach to patients with functional voice disorder. *Annals of Otology, Rhinology and Laryngology*, 91, 372–377.

KWEE, M. G. T. (1990). *Psychotherapy, Meditation and Health: A Cognitive–Behavioural Perspective*. London: East-West Publications.

KWEE, M. G. T. and LAZARUS, A. A. (1986). Multimodal therapy: The cognitive–behavioural tradition and beyond. In W. Dryden and W. Golden (eds) *Cognitive–Behavioural Approaches to Psychotherapy*. London: Harper and Row.

LUCHSINGER, R. and ARNOLD, G. E. (1965). *Voice, Speech and Language*. London: Constable.

MACCURTAIN, F. (1983). Vocal tract function in psychogenic voice disorders. *Proceedings of 19th Congress, International Association of Logopaedics and Phoniatrics*, pp.14–18. University of Utrecht, The Netherlands.

MARTIN, S. (1987) *Working with Dysphonics*. Oxfordshire: Winslow Press.

MARTIN, S. and DARNLEY, L. (1992). *The Voice Source Book*. Oxfordshire: Winslow Press.

MATHEWS, A. (1985). Anxiety states: A cognitive–behavioural approach. In B. P. Bradley and C. Thompson (eds) *Psychological Applications in Psychiatry*. Chichester: Wiley.

MEICHENBAUM, D. (1977). *Cognitive–Behaviour Modification*. New York: Plenum.

MEICHENBAUM, D. and GENEST, M. (1982). Cognitive behaviour modification: An integration of cognitive and behavioural methods. In F. H. Kanfer and A. P. Goldstein (eds) *Helping People Change*. New York: Pergamon.

MEICHENBAUM, D. H. and TURK, D. (1976). The cognitive–behavioural management of anxiety, anger and pain. In P. Davidson (ed.) *The Behavioural Management of Anxiety, Depression and Pain*. New York: Brunner/Mazel.

MITCHELL, L. (1987). *Simple Relaxation*. London: Murray.

MURPHY, A. T. (1964). *The Functional Voice Disorders*. Englewood Cliffs, NJ: Prentice-Hall.

NEIMEYER, R. A. (1986). Personal construct therapy. In W. Dryden and W. Golden (eds) *Cognitive–Behavioural Approaches to Psychotherapy*. London: Harper and Row.

NORDBY, V. J. and HALL, C. S. (1974). *A Guide to Psychologists and Their Concepts*. San Francisco: Freeman.

NOVACO, R. (1975). *Anger Control: The Development and Evaluation of an Experimental Treatment*. Lexington, MA: Lexington Books.

PERELLO, J. (1962). Dysphonies functionnelles: Phonoponos et Phonevrose. *Folia Phoniatrica*, 14, 150–205.

PERKINS, W. H. (1957). The challenge of functional disorders of voice. In L. E. Travis (ed.) *Handbook of Speech Pathology*. New York: Appleton/Century/Crofts.

PERKINS, W. H. (1973). Replacement of stuttering with normal speech: 1 Rationale. *Journal of Speech and Hearing Disorders*, 38, 283–294.

PUNT, N. (1979). *The Singer's and Actor's Throat*. London: Heinemann.

PURSER, H. (1982). *Psychology for Speech Therapists*. Leicester: British Psychological Society.

RACHMAN, S. J. and HODGSON, R. J. (1980). *Obsessions and Compulsions*. Englewood Cliffs, NJ: Prentice-Hall.

RATHUS, S. (1973). A 30-item schedule for assessing assertive behaviour. *Behaviour Therapy*, 4, 398–406.

ROGERS, C. R. (1951). *Client-Centred Therapy*. Boston: Houghton Mifflin.

ROGERS, C. R. (1961). *On Becoming a Person*. Boston: Houghton Mifflin.

ROTTER, J. B. (1966). Generalised expectancies for internal versus external control of reinforcement. *Psychological Monograph*, 80, 1, 1–28.

RUSH, A. J., BECK, A. T., KOVACS, M. and HOLLON, S. D. (1977). Comparative efficacy of cognitive therapy and pharmacotherapy in the treatment of depressed outpatients. *Cognitive Therapy and Research*, 1, 17–37.

RUTTER, M. (1975). *Maternal Deprivation Reassessed*. Harmondsworth: Penguin.

RYAN, B. P. and VAN KIRK, B. (1978). *Monterey Fluency Programme*. Palo Alto, CA: Monterey Learning Systems.

SALKOVSKIS, P. (1989). Obsessions and compulsions. In J. Scott, J. M. G. Williams, and A. T. Beck (eds) *Cognitive Therapy in Clinical Practice*. London: Routledge.

SCHWARTZ, R. M. (1986). The internal dialogue: On the asymmetry between positive and negative coping thoughts. *Cognitive Therapy and Research*, 10, 591–605.

SELIGMAN, M. E. D. (1975). *Helplessness*. San Francisco: Freeman.

SHEWELL, C. (1990). What the voice betrays. *Speech Therapy in Practice*. September, pp.15–16.

SHEWELL, C. (1992). *The Teaching of Inter-Personal Skills and Counselling to Speech and Language Therapy Students*. National Hospital's College of Speech Sciences, London. Unpublished.

SMITH, D. (1982). Trends in counselling and psychotherapy. *American Psychologist*, 37, 802–809.

SNAITH, P. (1981). *Clinical Neurosis*. Oxford: Oxford University Press.

SNAITH, R. P., CONSTANTOPOULOS, A. A., JARDINE, M. Y., AND MCGUFFIN, P. (1978). A clinical scale for the self-assessment of irritability. *British Journal of Psychiatry*, 132, 164–171.

STERN, R. and DRUMMOND, L. (1991). *The Practice of Behavioural and Cognitive Psychotherapy*. Cambridge: Cambridge University Press.

STEVENS, B. (1977). Voids, voids, voids – noddings. In John O. Stevens (ed.) *Gestalt Is*. New York: Bantam.

TURNBULL, J. (1987). Anxiety control training and its place in stuttering therapy. In C. Levy (ed.) *Stuttering Therapies: Practical Approaches*. London: Croom Helm.

VAN RIPER, C. (1973). *The Treatment of Stuttering*. Englewood Cliffs, NJ: Prentice-Hall.

VAN ROOD, Y. and GOULMY, E. (1990). Stress, relaxation and changes in the immune system. In M. G. T. Kwee (ed.) *Psychotherapy, Meditation and Health: A Cognitive–Behavioural Perspective*. London: East-West Publications.

WALLACE, R.K. and BENSON, H. (1972). The physiology of meditation. *Scientific American*, 226, 2, 84–90.

WEISHAAR, M. E. and BECK, A. T. (1986). Cognitive therapy. In W. Dryden and W. Golden (eds) *Cognitive–Behavioural Approaches to Psychotherapy*. London: Harper and Row.

WILLIAMS, J. M. G., WATTS, F. N., MACLEOD, C., MATHEWS, A. (1988). *Cognitive Psychology and Emotional Disorders*. Chichester: Wiley.

WILSON, P. H., SPENCE. S. H. and KAVANAGH, D. J. (1989). *Cognitive Behavioural Interviewing for Adult Disorders*. London: Routledge.

WOLPE, J. (1969). *The Practice of Behaviour Therapy*. New York: Pergamon Press.

YOUNG, J. E. and BROWN, G. (1990). *Schema Questionnaire*. Published by Cognitive Therapy Centre of New York, 111 West 88th St, New York, NY 10024, USA.

Author Index

Subject Index